A History of Disability

Corporealities: Discourses of Disability

David T. Mitchell and Sharon L. Snyder, editors

Books available in the series:

HENRI-JACQUES STIKER

A History of Disability

Translated by William Sayers

Ann Arbor

THE UNIVERSITY OF MICHIGAN PRESS

The publisher is grateful
for a partial subvention for translation from
the French Ministry of Culture.

English translation copyright © by the University of Michigan 1999
Originally published in 1997 by Éditions Dunod, Paris,
as *Corps infirmes et sociétés*,
a revised edition of the 1982 book by the same title,
published by Éditions Aubier Montaigne
Copyright © by Éditions Dunod 1997

2002   2001   2000   1999   4   3   2   1

A CIP catalog record for this book is available from the British Library.

Library of Congress Cataloging-in-Publication Data

Stiker, Henri-Jacques.
  [Corps infirmes et societes. English]
  A history of disability / Henri-Jacques Stiker ; translated by
William Sayers.
      p.   cm.—(Corporealities)
  Includes bibliographical references.
  ISBN 0-472-11063-2 (acid-free paper)
  ISBN 0-472-08626-X (acid-free paper)
    1. Handicapped—Social conditions.   I. Title.   II. Series.
HV1552 .S8413 1999
  362.4'09—dc21
                                          99-6494
                                            CIP

Contents

DAVID T. MITCHELL

Foreword

I first came upon the work of Henri-Jacques Stiker when he presented an overview of this book at a 1996 meeting of the Society for Disability Studies. As I sat in the audience listening to the English translation of his talk, I realized the history he offered went beyond previous work on disability and representation. Not only did disability represent a social construction of difference that marked disabled people as alien; the classification proved central to definitions of cultural value and imaginative investment. At the time the novelty of Stiker's approach struck me as significant in three specific ways: (1) the analysis of disability provided a window into the variability of the human body as a biological and historical entity; (2) the definition of disability was directly tied to the moral principles of Western cultures; (3) the pervasiveness of disability representation solidified the centrality of the category to historical and cultural analysis. Unlike other work on the history of disability produced prior to the mid-1990s,[1] Stiker's study provides neither a reassuring progressive trajectory nor a flat notion of negative and positive imagery. Instead, his work situates itself as a challenge to our own cultural progress narratives and political sophistication.

As a work of cultural anthropology, *A History of Disability* moves between numerous registers of academic inquiry. Stiker's method ranges from close readings of literary texts as exemplary of dominant myths to discussions of the etymology of disability terminology to medical taxonomies of specific conditions and test cases to an examination of current legislative initiatives. The book proceeds as an investigation into the reigning ideologies about disability in history and the language that serves as a medium for shaping cultural

attitudes. Because the "management" of disability is a preoccupation
of nearly every cultural domain—from literature to policy—the work
moves between these institutional perspectives in a Foucauldian effort to trace out the disciplinary construction of disability as a category of deviant exceptionality. Yet, unlike Foucault, Stiker works
against a view of history as a series of ruptures or breaks in the
construction of disability. Instead, he argues for a continuum of effects in which one epoch's beliefs continue to inform the practices of
succeeding generations. The multiple angles of approach into this
history of disability allows Stiker to approach his subject as a historical mosaic that provides a rounded and complex portrayal of disability as a powerful category of cultural analysis.

Like other French intellectuals in cultural studies, Stiker begins
with a psychoanalytic model. Yet the reader will not encounter in this
work any of the abstract theorization or deconstructive gimmickry of
much current theory. The book is written in a straightforward manner,
and a sense of urgency informs its prose. As a beginning principle,
Stiker posits that an encounter with disability inaugurates a break in
the observer's perceptual field—"a tear in our being that reveals [the
body's] open-endedness, its incompleteness, its precariousness." The
visceral nature of this "tear" reveals the extent of our investment in the
fantasy of the normal. Rather than accept a more dynamic foundation
upon which to base our notions of bodily function and appearance, the
upheaval of this encounter results from an assault upon our belief in
certainty in general and our desire to identify with a monolithic body
type in particular. Our cultural tutoring establishes biological integrity
as an unassailable expectation and a rite of passage into the world of
the normal. Our membership in the normal begins not only with the
fit of our own bodies into the dictates of the norm (one that is always
tenuous with or without a disability) but with our acceptance of the
norm as a controlling principle. For Stiker this belief proves not only
illusory but also the basis of social violence: "The love of difference or
the passion of similarity. The former—especially if it becomes socially
contagious (through education, cultural action, political action)—leads
to *human* life. The latter leads, in full-blown or latent form, to exploitation, repression, sacrifice, rejection."

This insistence upon the truth (and even desirability) of biological mutability—rather than physical stability or likeness—marks the ground zero of Stiker's politics. His work seeks simultaneously to demonstrate the presence of disability throughout Western history and to unmoor our collective fantasies in the "promise" of eradication or cure. Yet the dynamism of difference does not lead Stiker to a romanticized model that wishes away the complications of an embodied life. Instead, it seeks to substitute a more robust encounter with physical and cognitive difference as both a product of historical investments and a cleavage in our ideology of the desire for sameness. Rather than the classification of disability as abnormality or monstrosity, Stiker insists that the sign of the tragic that disability so often represents is not embedded in the organism but, rather, in the "conditions or the figurations in which we receive what is born or appears." With this formulation the symbolic becomes the determining medium of difference and socially inscribed meaning. To borrow from Simone de Beauvoir, one is not born a freak; one is made one.

A History of Disability provides a vast historical overview of key moments in the revision of disability's meanings. The fact that disability has refused to remain linguistically stable, in-and-of-itself, demonstrates the variability of the body and its socially generated interpretations. On the one hand, disabled populations remain segregated and marginal throughout history. On the other hand, cultures persist in creating difference into a paramount trope of the human condition. Stiker sets out to unravel this seeming contradiction that exists at the core of disability's symbolic classification. Beginning with the Talmud and the Old Testament, the author establishes that a surprising array of disabilities are recorded—the lame, blind, crippled, deaf, mute, contagious, mad—and a principle of exclusion invoked: the unsightly and sickly may not create or attend the rituals of the temple. Such a principle of exclusion situates itself in a generalized theory of hygiene: if one cannot satisfactorily differentiate between communicable diseases and genetic/environmental disorders, then any discernible blemish necessitates segregation. Disability designates the terms of a biological rejection and an obsession with dividing the pure from the impure.

For Stiker this Lévi-Straussian turn in Talmudic and Old Testament logic becomes an instance of public and sacral purification—disabilities signify both a risk to the social body and to religious sanctity. Thus commences the symbolic deployment of disability as a mediating figure between the unclean body and the purity of religious space. Disability as a synonym for the "unclean" enters into the Western tradition as a primary means of delineating between that which is earthly and dirty and that which is heavenly and clean. This equation excludes disabled people from religious practice but paradoxically places them within an ethical discourse of human value. What do people with disabilities reveal about God's will? Since that which God possesses must be, by definition, without blemish, disabilities made literal the evidence of the inherent imperfection of the human condition. Within this formulation disabilities resulted in social ostracization and in a tradition of representation that deploys disability as the master metaphor of humanity's essential corruption since the Fall.

While the New Testament seemingly breaks with this belief in disability as a sign of individual pollution, the healing of cripples still adheres to a desire for eradication—the temples are opened up by Jesus but only after the blemish has been miraculously removed. Stiker convincingly argues that the emphasis in either case highlights not the integral nature of disability to embodied life but, rather, the moral imperative behind their social integration. Christ disrupts the prior social mandate to segregate physical difference and transforms disabled people into a means by which Christians could best establish their religious commitments. The social conundrum of disability resides in this important distinction—the question of how to integrate disability into our cultural spaces (and thus our consciousness) implies a problem that still pervades Western systems of thought. Disability became an indicator of misfortune that must be integrated into a ritualized system of communal penitence, yet physical aberrancy remained outside definitions of human embodiment.

In formulating this problem, Stiker underlines a much more substantive conflict for contemporary disability studies scholars and the disability rights movement in general. The question of how to integrate people with disabilities into mainstream society sacrifices the concept of disability as an integral aspect of human nature. To request inclusion is to underscore one's desire for assimilation into a norm that supports the perception of disability as an alien or exceptional condition. A community's marginality is implicitly underscored by the request for inclusion itself. If disability can be theorized as essential to our definition of what constitutes the human, then the *integrable* must take a back seat to the *integral.* Stiker's historical analysis demonstrates that in each of the key epochs of Western thought—the classical era, the Middle Ages, the Renaissance, the Enlightenment, the Victorian age, the modern—that disability and disabled populations continue to surface as that which must be assimilated or made to disappear. The less visible physical and cognitive difference becomes, the more a society can pride itself upon its own illusory value as a human(e) collectivity. The "success" of integration can be based upon a variety of assimilation strategies, from legislative policies to segregation to eradication, but Stiker argues that there is a disturbing ideology underwriting each action along this continuum—the social ideal of erasure.

A *History of Disability* argues that, ironically, a professed will to integration characterizes most epochs' treatment of people with disabilities, yet none to this point in history has committed themselves to a belief in the "naturalness" of physical and cognitive differences to the normative human condition. Rather than expending efforts to physically or rhetorically remove disability from public purview, an acceptance of disability would result in the development of more flexible social systems, values, and expectations. Instead, as Stiker demonstrates, all periods evidence strategies for making disabled people over in the image of the norms of the day. For the ancient Athenians people with disabilities were provided with public funds to sustain themselves like their fellow able-bodied citizens; in the Middle Ages friars from the mendicant orders sought to live among the disabled and outcast as a sign of their commitment to the "poor and unfortunate"; the fourteenth-century ethic of charity transformed disabled people into needy objects through whom the rich could achieve salvation; Renaissance courts provided a space for fools and dwarves to satirize the pretensions of the ruling classes; the advent of medical institutions discarded demonology as a root cause of disabilities but interned the "unfit" in order to promote the rule of order; the late eighteenth century presided over the birth of educational facilities as a way to "raise up and restore" disabled people to a level of acceptable functionality; the nineteenth-century discourse of rehabilitation situated disability as a "lack to be filled" by medical correction and technology. In each case disabled populations are linguistically transformed by a value-laden designation that determined their placement within a preordained social order.

Significantly, Stiker reserves his fiercest critique for the twentieth century. Founded upon a principle of rehabilitation in which all differences can be ultimately obliterated with prosthetics, exercise regimes, medical interventions, and the cultivation of the disabled individual's desire for assimilation to the norm, the twentieth century has single-mindedly committed itself to its own integrationist ideal. While nineteenth-century medical discourses of restoration still abound, our century forwards legislative initiatives seeking to "level the playing field" between disabled and nondisabled. According to Stiker, this rehabilitative approach "marks the appearance of a culture that attempts to complete the act of identification, of making identical." The rhetoric of sameness dominates the twentieth century by vehemently promoting the erasure of differences as its ultimate goal—we are all essentially the same and therefore equal. The promise to restore an individual back into the fold of "normal" life simultaneously reasserts the notions of abnormality and normalcy. While Stiker does not deny that access to rights and equal opportunities is a necessary precursor of social participation and influence, he does argue that "making alterity disappear" serves as little more than a contemporary policy gloss upon the realities of disabled lives. Our rhetoric extols the desirability of a fully integrated society while overlooking the persistence of widespread "disparities, contradictions, and roughness [that] remain." To elide our engagement with the reality of difference by promoting an ambiguous language of civil(ized) homogeneity becomes tantamount to denying disability the uniqueness of its demands upon the individual and sociality alike.

For scholars of disability this is provocative stuff and requires us to apply a more exacting scrutiny to demands for equal rights and "inclusion." While some readers may find Stiker's argument politically insensitive to recent policy "breakthroughs" such as the Americans with Disabilities Act (this book was originally published in 1982), the challenge of his arguments remain salient. While legislation has offered a degree of legal recourse to those seeking protection and reparation from discrimination, the ADA has been narrowly interpreted by the courts and successfully employed by a host of questionable causes opportunistically riding beneath the banner of disability. As Stiker points out, the rhetoric of integration often pays lip service to the ideal of equality. Legislation is concerned only that disabled people pass the threshold to invisibility. We reference the ADA as an indicator of our society's commitment to social justice while failing to achieve demonstrable evidence of its successful implementation.

Integration into the norm becomes the hurdle that we must clear, and those who fail to make it are quickly left behind. Disability requires adaptation, and we fool ourselves if we believe our buildings and policies will be expected to change more than the individuals who must access them. Stiker argues that an emphasis upon the integral (rather than the integrable) nature of disability to human existence would result in the reconceptualization of the workday itself or expectations of productivity based upon the divergent capacities of the individual. Since all people fear their inevitable transition into disability, why see personal human history only diachronically with disability at the end of human narrative, when it could be seen synchronically as everywhere represented whether as a consequence of birth, accident, or age? Once we recognize that human capacities vary greatly from one another and that those differences mark the dynamic essence of what it means to be human, cultures can begin to adapt to the value of individual differences rather than differentiate between the value of individuals.

NOTE

1. Since the mid-1990s there have been several books published on the history of disability and representation: Lennard Davis, *Enforcing Normalcy: Disability, Deafness, and the Body* (London: Verso, 1995), Rosemarie Garland Thomson, *Extraordinary Bodies: Figuring Physical*

Disability in American Culture and Literature (New York: Columbia University Press, 1997), and David Mitchell and Sharon Snyder, *The Body and Physical Difference: Discourses of Disability* (Ann Arbor: University of Michigan Press, 1997). Like Stiker's book, these studies forward analyses of disability as a complex category of cultural and literary representation. The publication of *A History of Disability* marks the first time Stiker's work has been published in English.

WILLIAM SAYERS

Translator's Note

If the Italian maxim "traddutore tradditore" (the translator is a traitor) continues to be valid, we should expect few notes from translators, since treason seldom seeks publicity. Yet some texts and the cultures from which they spring will be so remote from the contemporary reader as to be nearly unviable in another language without some explanatory apparatus. With works closer in time and cultural space, one could argue that the translator's notes undermine translation itself by always calling attention to its inadequacies. The authority of the authorial voice is invalidated, as the translator has the superior, condescending last word. Every translator's choice, every linguistic equivalence that is established, could, in principle, become the subject of comment and thereby of justification, until the notes threaten the body of the work itself in a fantastic scenario from Borges or Nabokov, where the gloss swallows the word.

With this one exception there are no translator's notes to the English version of Henri-Jacques Stiker's *Corps infirmes et sociétés.* The author himself displays the translator's consciousness of how language renews itself, how, in a given field, one term succeeds another, with a semantic charge, a valence in public discourse, that may be intended as more positive or more negative, or simply more neutral, than those preceding. But, as concerns the pursuit of impartiality, the reiterated effort is often in vain. The newly minted term fits and wears poorly and is gradually debased when social reality and its informing mental representations fail to change in accord with the optimistic assumption of new terminology. As the succession in words for race, ethnicity, and culture illustrate, the seemingly neutral term can quickly be given a wash of emotion and prejudice and, except for its phonological exoskeleton, becomes the word it replaced.

These observations, none particularly new, bear on the latter part of Stiker's book in two important ways. The notion of remedial social intervention in the face of disability—rehabilitation—was linguistically configured in various ways in French in the course of the late nineteenth and early twentieth centuries. The author's discussion tracks several such terms closely, most of which have an English cognate and superficial equivalent, for example, *réadaptation*, "readaptation." But these English words, particularly when addressing disability, have not at all had the same history as their French counterparts, displaying neither their sequence in general usage nor their relative frequency nor their shifting affective colorations. To keep the reader's focus on the history of the French words, despite the distraction of the differing histories of the English translations, the French term is often given in the text when initially discussed and is occasionally recalled later, as appropriate. So much for the vocabulary of rehabilitation.

More important, the concept and linguistic dress of disability itself are no less immune to such change. Stiker is eloquent on the subject of the negative prefixes, *dis-*, *im-*, *in-*, *non-*, *un-*, that have been part of so much terminology and on the various recent efforts to find a lexicon for disability that does not immediately call up notions of deficiency rather than difference. What strikes the translator, shuttling between languages, is that early this century, when French sought to renew itself lexically to readdress disability, it seemed to lack the inherent will to create from its own resources. Perhaps French society, government agencies, and organizations were open to the influence of perceived social advances abroad as they sought to reconfigure disability mentally and linguistically. Or the loan of the English word *handicap* may have been a simple expedient, a quick fix from a language that was affecting French in so many others areas of culture and technology. Language history is full of ironies; *handicap* continues in French (albeit threatened), when its vogue in English is over, the ground having been ceded to *disability*—whose own future is, of course, not secure. In the translation from French *infirme* and *handicapé* have both been translated as *disabled.*

Yet, in the ongoing play of texts and languages with authors and readers, even the traitorous translator may not have the last word. In the wake of translation come copyediting and marketing. An imagined future readership becomes the final arbiter of acceptable linguistic usage. But, in closing, back to basics: what we are now prepared to read in English will be at some remove from its French original, just as the historical texts cited in Stiker's book will have had their own lexicon of disability, very likely with associations and connotations beyond our recovery and outside present norms of ethics and taste.

HENRI-JACQUES STIKER

Preface to the 1997 Edition

Rereading oneself is a trial, a matter of putting oneself to the test again. The reprinting of a book fifteen years after its first appearance certainly proves that there is a still a demand. But on the other hand, just how solid is what was proposed back then? Each chapter, even each statement of this work, would entail extended research. The elliptical character of this essay, which covers more than twenty centuries, is evident. This imposes a choice: to leave the book in its present state, counting on the advantages of brevity, or to lengthen it. But lengthening it would have been an endless process, not so much to account for the studies that have been published in the last decade and a half, important as they are in many ways, as to fill in the gaps that have been left unaddressed by others. Indeed, if the history of certain disabilities, and of what impinges on them, has advanced in recent years (mental retardation, deafness, blindness, special education, vocational rehabilitation, to take only a few examples), if sociological and psychoanalytical approaches have equipped us to penetrate more deeply into social constructions or institutional systems, the anthropology of disability has scarcely progressed. In the face of the fear of rewriting a book to double, triple, or quadruple its original length—which would have been contrary to the demand for a reprinting—I have left my text from 1982 as it is without adding other correctives than in matters of detail and in the conclusion and afterword, always uncertain areas when one risks putting forth one's own ideas. In these two places I shall explain my current position.

While leaving the text more or less unchanged, I have, however, added or expanded many footnotes, the one process compensating for

the other, at least in part. In the present state of studies of the history
and anthropology of disability these references will serve in place of
discursive text, and my brief mentions can serve as markers of avenues
for future research.

But one question has not stopped plaguing me. My effort remains
isolated. I have not stimulated the debate that I had expected, although
some academics such as Michelle Perrot, Alain Corbin, and Antoine
Prost have recognized the importance of this field. Even if the weaknesses of my book were faulted, it remains distressing that no university
chair in history, no program in anthropology, has been devoted to this
dimension of society. At least not in France. The French translation of
Robert Murphy's book *The Body Silent* is one of the rare studies of
disability that made its way into an editorial series in the human sciences. The author is American, and he was already disabled when he
wrote it. *Disability,* a generic term for the moment, just like *sexuality,
power,* or *barter,* is a constant phenomenon that has given rise to, or has
entered into, many cultural systems. Why this lack of attention on the
part of researchers and teachers in the human sciences? Today, to give
greater acuity to this question, 5 percent of the French population and
10 percent of the world population are directly affected by a disability,
while the total public outlay in this area in France is more than one
hundred and fifty billion francs annually (approx. $25 billion), a little
less than 2 percent of the gross national product. Seen from every side,
the subject appears rich—but thinkers shy away from it. Can it be the
fundamental unease deep within us when faced with deformed bodies
and troubled minds? Yet we have not failed to become interested in
insanity, mental illness, and more recently AIDS. In our time, it is true,
the public forum is occupied by genetic illnesses but with a view to
relating them to biology and medicine as objects of research. The social
sciences continue to ignore them. Is it because they are only too content
to have them eradicated and thus not to have to bother with them? Or is
it that service organizations and the medical establishment are reluctant
to appeal to these so-called social sciences? Other hypotheses could also
be formulated, without any doubt. But asking the question is not the
same thing as answering it. Who, in the scientific domain, will agree to
debate the topic?

While I wait, I have the great satisfaction of noting that the persons directly or indirectly concerned have given evidence of a heightened desire to understand past and present systems of thought and practice, systems of which they are the heirs or tributaries. I hope that these people will find grist for their mills in the pages that follow, reedited on the initiative of the Association of Paralytics of France and released in France by a publishing house that is clearly attentive to their concerns. As for my academic colleagues, I shall try in the future to find the ways and means to convince them.

1

Introduction

I have been thinking for a long time now about the proper way to write about the subject of these pages. The subject is unambiguous as concerns the degree of intelligibility I am looking for: the social and cultural ways of viewing—and of dealing with—what we so imprecisely call disability. This inquiry must be conducted with rigor. But we cannot talk of what relates to suffering in the way we dissect ancient myths or dispute Brownian effects. This is not so much because of moral scruple or a sentimental sense of propriety—all matters worthy of the greatest attention—but primarily because affectivity, "the heart" as we say, can never be separated from the observations that we make, from the analysis that we undertake, and because we assume responsibility with the publication of research.

Whoever addresses disability (the valence of this concept is of no matter for the moment) is engaged in its study in a personal capacity, even if it is only through texts. But even more so if one is close to its acute, living difficulty. Certain affective pre-apprehensions always accompany our efforts to understand its psychological or physical effect and the social space that surrounds and circumscribes it.

The issue of responsibility is likewise implicated in the study of disability. People struck by disability, and their circle of family and friends, are among us . . . and among our readers. Every effort at theorizing also enters into a relational context, into a communication. Certainly, intellectual inquiry, by virtue of its particular nature, and the play of language that is proper to it, ought to enjoy independence and should not have to please or displease, offend or flatter. Nor should it have to justify the appropriateness or timing of its statements.

But the very rigor that orders intellectual inquiry and every hypothesis that makes it possible require that it accept its limitations and that it identify the domain where it will not penetrate. No investigation has the right to present its results as the totality, as complete; Western intelligence has too long exploited this pretension and has too often presumed that knowledge was finite and fully attainable. Exclusionary thought, which is not a thing of the past,[1] mutilates the intelligence. The solidity of a proof, the potential of a line of thought, along with the conviction to which they lead, are not contrary to a sense of limit, in short, to a sense of humor. Thus, respect for our intended readership—a respect that is not outmoded—is part of the approach, and not simply part of the accompanying ethics. Responsibility is tied to intelligibility, even prior to being an ethical requirement.

For these two quite precise reasons—the inevitably affective position of the researcher, the necessarily limited situation of the discourse—I will not abstain from making a personal disclosure before the developments that follow, provided the narrow-minded don't object.

At the risk of being dismissed even before being read, I shall begin by being outraged. That's right, outraged: at seeing the two implications of research that I have identified so often disregarded. When the parents of autistic children[2] come to psychiatrists who have a smattering of psychoanalysis and are ensconced in their medical institutions, they have no need, in the first instance, to have bits and pieces of theoretical discussions thrown in their faces. As if these were to illustrate a conceptual framework that, moreover, only poorly camouflages the ignorance and affective poverty of these practitioners. When persons confined to a wheelchair or crippled by traumatic aftereffects come before the authorities responsible for settling their cases[3] in order to clear the way to some few rights, there is no need for them to feel that they are objects of rivalry among agencies, as if they were stakes in a game of social strategy, theorized or still theorizable, that scarcely conceals the nonchalance of these operators of the bureaucratic machinery.

A long list of situations could be recited, as you can easily imagine. They all come down to the neglect of certain levels of analysis in favor of an unwarranted projection or a legitimate elaboration that come from some other source. This is why I want to say up front what, as a consequence of the demands of methodology, I will forget in what follows (except at certain select moments!). To what, in the mental and/or physical order of things, am I referred by the existence of these multiple diminutions or insufficiencies: *mal-formation, dis-ability, de-bility, im-potence,* etc? All these words, curiously negative (negating what?), evoke a fear. At its lowest level, or on its surface if you like, this fear produces an almost visceral reaction to the disruption that has been caused. We organize the world—that is, space and time and, within these, social roles, cultural paths, ways of living, moving about, getting to work, styles of communication, and habits of leisure—for a kind of average person, designated normal. This is a world that the person who cannot, or can no longer, move there comfortably threatens to modify and remake. The first fear is a discomfort, a kind of strain that is imposed by the being who is no longer located within our familiar norms. This first fear is quickly aggravated when we confront the transformations that follow its admission: our life shatters, our plans collapse, and, beyond us as individuals, the various social organizations appear rigid, closed, hostile—they would have to be blown apart. In us, or around us, the onset of a disability creates a disorganization that is both concrete and social. But from this vantage point we perceive yet another disorganization, much deeper and more painful: the disorganization of our acquired understandings, of our established values.

Mental disorganization: why all these misfortunes? How do they occur? How could this happen to *me?* My image of myself, constructed with effort to live, to survive, to face others—with its inevitable share of masks and pretenses, with the no less inevitable and necessary repressions—blurs, trembles, even cracks. I thought I was like this . . . and look what I've become! I thought people saw me like that . . . and look how I'll seem now! I thought myself charged with life, rich in potential . . . and look what I've produced! I admired the imminent in my life . . . and now it's weakened and at times repellent, or hostile. I saw the world in a certain way, along with society and other people, and now they are completely different: much more vulnerable, much more ill willed, and at times much more unexpected or even much better. Everything changes place; everyone changes roles. All realities disclose an unedited other side. I have to start all over again . . . and in solitude, even if I am surrounded. Because it is *my* vision that is being wiped out—with its illusions and its reference points—and no one can understand or reconstruct it for me. Disorganization of what I call my values. We all have values—whatever we call them—even the most skeptical, the most despairing, the most lucid, the most philosophical, the most disenchanted of us. Friendships, acquaintanceships, even those that were sincere and rewarding, come undone. Our loves—even if we thought them without end—bend and sometimes break. Personal confidences are lost. Ideals and facile hopes erode. And then, when hope is reborn, when the taste for life returns, when new relationships are formed, it is not without a bitter smile that I hear again talk of happiness or the announcement of brighter futures. Nothing, nothing, is left but a vague and cold tension not to fall apart. I face my fear.

But the fear that I feel is an ancestral one, for in the end it is the fear of fault. Somewhere in me there lies a culpability, and I am made to feel it acutely. Somewhere in the world of the living, or in the universe, something is responsible for the catastrophe that happens to me or that I see strike another. People have never felt comfortable with what appears deformed, spoiled, broken. Is it because they never knew whose fault it was? Yet there is no lack of explanations for misfortune and suffering! But all the philosophers and theologians in the world have never exorcized this special treatment except by underlining it with their very explanations. If it is a consequence of sin . . . then I am more of a victim than others and doubtless more guilty in one sense or another. If it is fate, then I am even more rejected, and the object of some mystifying condemnation. If it is society, I am even more of a pariah, since I know that society is ruthless. If it is the law of the majority, I am the exception, fit only for the scrap heap. If it's my genes, then I am a plague carrier. If it's my psychological attitude, my unconscious behavior, I'm ready for therapy in perpetuity. If it is my own irresponsible or reckless conduct, I am entirely to blame. I am ringed in by explanations on every side. Need I look for a new one? Perhaps not an explanation but an assessment. Isn't the first question, the one that misfortune itself causes us to forget, this one: why is disability called "dis-ability"? Why are those who are born or become different referred to by all these various names? Why so many categories? Why even such dramatics in the face of what happens . . . so often, and which can happen to any of us? Clearly, because human life is not ready to accept "that," because society is not organized for "that," because exceptional measures and procedures are always called for, because we have to turn to specialized persons and institutions (and how could we do otherwise?), and so on. But, in a more fundamental way, where does that huge exercise in naming come from, that labeling that circumscribes one kind of reality (the *disability* in today's vocabulary) and makes us feel it all the more and be more afraid of it? Otherwise, it is well-known, often experienced, always dreaded, the moment when the doctor, the relative, the social worker, declares, "It's . . ." It's "autism," it's "paraplegia," it's "serious retardation." In short, a bit like the plague or consumption in the past and cancer today. The "thing" is there, and the condemnation falls.

But when we name, we point up a *difference.* I am Jacques, and so I am neither Pierre nor Paul. It is the wonderful clarity of the opening books of the Bible in which God distinguishes, separates, differentiates by naming, to the point where to create is to separate;[4] we also see one being (Eve) come out of another (Adam) but affirmed as Difference even in the name that is cried out.

Actually, it is no accident that I am thinking of this biblical passage at this point. Indeed, man and woman do constitute a difference: the one is not the other; the other is not the one. Sex separates, differentiates. But here the difference is *recognized* as soon as it is stated: this Eve, henceforth distant, is declared at the same time "the flesh of his flesh and the bones of his bones" by Adam. And even if the history of relations between man and woman is the history of the exclusion of woman by man in many domains—a sad outcome in light of the myth of Genesis—this difference has always been accepted and experienced and integrated by the force of circumstances. Certainly, woman has always frightened man—and has always made him feel what he doesn't have. Her difference makes possible gestation and birth! Man has always terrified woman—and attracted her, often tragically—man who seems to have a mysterious affinity with war. "The war of the sexes" is not a vain phrase, and there is a long-time loser in the affair, namely woman. But the alliance is obligatory and the difference—whether worrisome, patched over, or erased by an infinite number of systems—remains no less constraining, inevitable, socialized, organized.

When we put a name on the difference represented by a being who is out of the ordinary, it is no longer the creative gesture that we imitate (to distinguish in order to create a whole!), it is no longer Adam's admiring cry that we repeat (the different, equal . . . and similar!), it is no longer even the awkward but ongoing history of a difference, fertile even though forced, which we re-inaugurate. It is the DIFFERENCE, untamed and unshared, that we designate; a difference without circumstance, without site; a raw difference that cannot be relegated somewhere, against which we must *protect ourselves*, a difference that generates a dark terror. We are suddenly faced with an unaccustomed bit of the *real*. This reality is too singular to be borne. What I thought I knew well—me, the other—what I had confidence in, what reassured me, is revealed as completely different. An unexpected, invisible aspect of reality looms up here and now, and suddenly constitutes a threat *without appeal;* there is an "accidental eruption of the real, that is, of a reality both undesirable and until then warded off by a set of seemingly resistant, solid, and proven mental constructions."[5] This is what we call a catastrophe. A catastrophe ensues from the fact that I didn't know reality could give birth to "that." I had built myself a world where I had not anticipated that such a difference, such a particularity, could spring out. In other words, alterity has surfaced from under a difference that cannot be situated.

Georges Canguilhem says the same thing, although in a more intellectual register, at the beginning of an article that I cannot resist citing at some length:

> The existence of monsters calls into question life in its capacity to teach us order. This questioning is immediate, no matter how long our prior confidence may have been, no matter how solid may have been our habit of seeing roses bloom on rose bushes,

tadpoles change into frogs, mares suckle colts and, in general fashion, of seeing like engender like. All that is needed is one loss of this confidence, one morphological lapse, one specific appearance of equivocation, and a radical fear seizes us. Fear? that I understand, you will say, but why radical? Because we are living beings, real effects of the laws of life, and the eventual causes of life in our turn. A failure on the part of life concerns us doubly because a failure could have afflicted us and a failure could come about through us. It is only because humans are living creatures that a morphological mistake is, to our living eyes, a monster. Suppose that we were pure reason, pure intellectual machines that observed, calculated and summed up, and thus inert and indifferent to the events that made us think: the monster would only be other than the same, of an order other than the most probable order.[6]

In France these days the expression *refus de la différence* (denial of the difference) has been overworked and trivialized to the point of being a publicity catchword. But a disability, even one that people call mild (with a questionable relativism, for everything depends on what you feel), does subject us to a great fear, disconcerting and isolated, to a prodigious act of negation. At this point we start by denying it, by becoming obsessive, by experiencing everything as a function of the fright and the discomfort that it causes, by delimiting and closing it in. Above all, the difference must not become contagious. We can't do anything about it . . . it has to be forgotten; but like a nightmare it lives within us from that time on. Then, social agencies have to intervene, to provide relief. To help us face up to it, as they say. Of course, but first of all to rid us of it, in a real or *symbolic* way, it all depends, or both at the same time. This is also the reason why it must be stated that we do not distinguish spontaneously the degrees and the disparities; aberration, whether it be mental, psychological, or physical, leads to the same fear and the same rejection. Moreover, within that difference that is disability, it is a difficult task to succeed in differentiating without accepting some differences in order better to exclude others. All the efforts—and I don't discredit any—to gain ground, to overcome fear in the face of this or that form of deformity, to live with it and make it live, always leave somewhere a terror and a *radical* loss of memory as one of the manifestations of terror. At every level, even among those who are designated disabled, the same denials recur. Each of us has a disabled other who cannot be acknowledged.

It should be noted that fear of the abnormal is not, as one might believe, to be confused with that of disease. The dividing line is not always sharp, even from an objective point of view. Mental and social categories of defect and disease have varied, we admit, but however the boundary is drawn in various periods and societies there is always a distinction. Disease, because of the fear of contagion, can approximate a defect. The case of lepers at various times in history illustrates the point. But the fear of disease is tied to the fear of death. I won't cry over my sick son who risks dying in at all the same way I will over my retarded or paralyzed child. Feelings of anguish don't all have the same reasons. The fear of an ending or of seeing disappear those who are close to us does not have the confrontation of difference as its motivation; it is the terror of the void and the terror of losing what makes us live, what our spiritual life clings to (in ways that may, admittedly, be pathological). The fear of death, affecting all life, does call humanity into question and, more narrowly, my identity. This fear, however, does not cast doubt on me as an individual and normal human being. Disability, on the other hand, strikes me in that very elementary and perhaps unsophisticated need not to be exiled, misunderstood, strange and a stranger, in my own eyes at first, then in the eyes of others.[7]

But disease, death, and monstrosity certainly come together at one point: in the desire to kill. We should not hide from the fact that major disability, especially mental, generates such an urge to make it disappear that it must be called by its name. In embryonic form the desire to kill, to see dead, is extended to all those who are stricken. The practice in antiquity of doing away with deformed children originates in a sense of eugenics, in the will for a pure race, and thus reveals what lies in the human heart. Let's not have any illusions; we carry within ourselves the urges to kill, because death and fear, like aggression, have their roots there.[8] It is obvious that this violence toward the different resolves itself in other ways than in the elimination of the disabled, thanks to socialization, with its rules, its prohibitions, and its institutions. Social systems are more or less murderous, that is, more or less astute in diverting and channeling spontaneous, savage violence—hence the importance of the study of these systems, which the present book undertakes. We must constantly remind ourselves of these desires, urges, and fears buried within us, which hide from and elude our clear consciousness but which are always alive and active.

Thus, it is the peculiarity represented by malformation or deformation that provokes a kind of panic both internal and public. And this feeling of not being like the others prompts the most contradictory behavior; we can profit by it to grant ourselves favors, attentions, and rights that only serve to highlight our weakness and to attach blame to others as well; we can withdraw, hide, be ashamed, and reinforce our solitude, even create it; we can demand of ourselves and of others that the disability fill the whole horizon, in order to deny, in retribution, the right to life of the able and healthy. The aggressiveness and the aggressions that disability provokes are multiform and include both masochism and sadism. This can often be a quite legitimate defense in the face of the condemnation of our surroundings, a condemnation that is also polyvalent. All this can be transformed into a rational program of support and struggle in a society in which all the machinery and customs are prejudicial and constraining for the disabled. Whether the character of these battles is paternalistic, trade unionist, political, or simply humanitarian—and all do not have the same status and value, as we shall see in the following—they will never hide, no more than will other patterns of behavior, the unease and the deep, fundamental disorientation that must also be accounted for, that must be taken into account at every moment.

I will not allow this stock of very specific anguish the spurious outlet of a moral or sociological justification. But I do believe that it is rooted in the fear of the different,[9] for we desire similarity, and, even more, we desire identicalness. Our desire to desire like others, to be and to have like others,[10] the strength, almost instinctive, to appropriate and exploit another person, his desires or her goods, the enormous need to imitate, to engage unceasingly in pantomimes—all these old mechanisms are just so many secular, archaic barriers to accepting what appears as monstrosity. The defect, somatic and mental, distances us too much from our reactions of conformity, from our love of the same. Is there a remedy for this?

To begin with, let us admit the very *primordial* function that the disabled fill. Like the child for the adult, like woman for man (and vice versa), they are proof of the inadequacy of what we would like to see established as references and norm. They are the tear in our being that reveals its open-endedness, its incompleteness, its precariousness. Because of that, because of that difference, they can, like children and women, be considered expiatory victims, scapegoats. But they prevent human society from setting up health, vigor, strength, cleverness, and intelligence as rights and as models to be imitated. They are the thorn in the side of the social group that prevents the folly of certainty and of identification with a single model. There is no mistaking it: the folly of the fit is exposed by the Down's syndrome child, the woman without arms, the worker in a wheelchair.

Much as we must put our energy into proclaiming this function for disability, we must just as necessarily avoid asserting its social and spiritual necessity. We cannot resurrect an idea that has dominated the centuries: the poor are necessary for the rich to be converted (and to become charitable!). I in no way assert the indispensable and beneficial character of disability. But I do say that such difference, when it arises, plays a balancing and warning role unlike any other. Our assurances and mimetic references, our normativized visions lose their standing. Not to overelaborate at this point, let me offer as moral fable the short English film that ran on television quite some time ago, which shows an everyday world organized and built for human beings who are all in wheelchairs. Then the day comes when a man is born, able to stand on his own two legs. He bumps into the transoms of doorways, gets around with difficulty on ramps not meant for walking, and so on. Then a series of malformations of this kind appears. Specialized associations for remedial education, retraining, accessibility issues, are consequently created, of course without anyone thinking about changing the basic assumptions of this society of the legless.

So I will simply say, although it amounts to rebellion and a near-utopia: let's love the difference. The spirituality—I'll risk the word—to which all aberration leads us, physical as well as mental (and the two are really only one), is actually quite simple: live everyday life as an everyday thing, with and in the presence of special, specific human beings who are our disabled equals. Of course, this is revolt because it takes back to the drawing board the whole enormous, vast, imposing specialized social organization: associations at the legislative level, public agencies at the family level. And a near-utopia since social constructs, patterns of thought, and especially the family dramas *are there.* Yes, dramas; you will admit that in many situations, at many moments, in many places, it happens that this "living with" is intolerable, harmful for the person struck by impairment and for the others. Finally, isn't it fresh folly to deny the utility, the inevitability, the necessity of the vast number of arrangements and institutions whose benefits are patent, whose results striking, whose relief irreplaceable? How misunderstood I would be if it were thought that I were pretentiously deleting with a single pen stroke these indispensable and beneficial activities—rather than choose among them! I don't have a problem with all of that, rather with everything that *can* make us forget, everything that can make us give up, everything that doesn't say well enough what ought to animate it all. I've written *spirituality* (although the word is hard to use well) in order to situate myself, in this introductory chapter to my work, above or beyond the discussion of institutions. It is our heart, that is, whatever determines the meaning of our actions, whatever gives direction to our existence, the place where we can be without lies or distortions, the inaugural point of our lives, that I address. Whatever you do, whichever battle you fight, whichever course of action you attempt, with what are you going to inform it all? The love of difference or the passion for similarity? The former—especially if it becomes socially contagious (through education, cultural action, political action)—leads to *human* life. The latter leads, in full-blown or latent form, to exploitation, repression, sacrifice, rejection. Yes or no, can we live together in fundamental mutual recognition, or must we exclude one another?

So that this question doesn't remain simple moralizing, the conditions for responding to it should be briefly clarified. Not to convince another to be like ourselves and not to force another to conform to a

model presupposes that we accept the real, which generates difference and singularity. In turn, accepting what is given presupposes,
first, an effort to know. These would then be preconditions for a reconciliation that is not just false egalitarianism: to learn that difference is
not an exception, not a monstrosity, but something that happens in the
natural course of things. But you will see on every side that this
understanding no more suffices to banish the fear of disability than
does science to eliminate racism by demystifying the fable of the
inferiority of certain races. We must then inscribe in our cultural
models a view of difference as the law of the real. It is a matter of
stating and restating, first of all to children throughout their education, that it is inscribed in the human universe to value the differences
it engenders and of which it is also a product. To prevent someone
from imposing the law of the identical, from proclaiming his identity as
unique, there is only one recourse beyond the ethical imperative, and
that is to make it a part of our culture.

Having said that—in particular in a phrase like "the law of the
real"—it is not my intention to reintroduce a naturalist viewpoint. To
announce that difference is the law of the real is the same as saying that
the real is only a succession of disparities and mutations. If the natural is
what differs, it is no longer the natural of old, and then the words hardly
matter. The law of the real appears as antinature, that is, far from
asserting a fixity, it causes diversity. I don't claim that disability, which
occurs in the same way as sex, build, and skin color, is a natural given in
the sense in which that suggests an idea of destiny. Naturalism, in this
domain, belongs to the workings of liberalism, as we shall see. I simply
believe that disability happens to humanity and that there are no
grounds for conceiving of it as an aberration. Life and biology have their
share of risks, as does life in society. No blind submission is implied
here; the struggle against disability and its causes is no less fierce, but,
instead of presenting it as an anomaly or as an abnormality, I conceive of
it in the first place as a reality. For me the tragic is not situated as for the
Greeks in what is born and appears; it lies in the conditions and the
figurations in which we receive what is born and appears. The tragic will
always be sufficiently present; let's not extend it, in some kind of morbid
cult, beyond the sites where it arises. If we do not submit to this reality,

the generator of differences, among which is disability, we will be imposing the law of the able, and then why not the law of the abler among the able, and finally why not the law of the ablest of all? After all, the eugenics movement was one of the bases of Nazism. The logic here is terrifying. As luck would have it, we are not rigorously logical—but, in its essence, every rejection of difference is totalitarian and dictatorial, and gentle ways have often been preferred to brutal ones.

Why, now, am I about to undertake a demanding work on the history of social modes of behavior toward the out of the ordinary?

Even if it were true that aggression toward difference has *at all times* been at the core of the problem (not stated in the foregoing, since the author was at issue there), it would still be necessary to know how and to what degree various societies have practiced such aggression. On which coordinate, on which scale, is *our* society in relation to others? The spirituality of which I spoke could never, in any way, be a substitute for clarity of vision and action, whatever its *determining* power may be. Systems that have tried to deny and/or live the difference are numerous and varied. Without this historical diffraction, what could we know about disability, how could we *situate* it, which possibilities and which pitfalls would we be capable of charting?

A personal decision, in relation to a life experience—even if this experience resonates in a multitude of other individuals—cannot lead to understanding and praxis unless it can be verified against historically known behaviors. To skimp on an examination of the mediating constructions and linkages that this age-old problem has encountered would be the same as saying next to nothing about it; the general nature of the commentary would dilute the problem. Tracing the ways in which different communities and cultures have addressed and managed the question is to follow human debate and see the numerous faces of a problem that is still before us. We illuminate a question better by following its development through time than by trying to fix it in a false eternal moment. Can we take a photograph of all the photos and a photograph of all the movements of our child? We know her better by looking at her often and under differing circumstances than by trying to capture her in so privileged a fashion that it becomes an illusion.

Michel Foucault has demonstrated, throughout the history of systems of thought (the clinic, the prison, sexuality, etc.)—from the hard evidence, if I may use the phrase—that a dominant point of view is not possible. There is no history of thought outside the history of *systems* of thought. There is no speech outside systems of languages. There is no spirituality outside received spiritual frameworks. There is no disability, no disabled, outside precise social and cultural constructions; there is no attitude toward disability outside a series of societal references and constructs. Disability has not always been *seen* in the same way. If I made the foregoing personal remarks, it is not by virtue of a transhistorical view but as a function of a set of perceptions that live within me and come to me, more than I dominate and live within them. I, myself, cannot speak for the Chinese of the second century of our era, the Aztec of an earlier epoch, the African from the time of Jesus, or the caveman; I can only, modestly, try to understand (where possible) *how* these different persons were situated and, when asked, say what seem to be the consequences for me, for us, in our very limited present world. There really is no solution to the problem of continuity between this introductory chapter, which does not directly address the subject of research, and the body of this book, which does not directly address the person invaded by his present suffering. I wanted to begin by speaking of my attitude, out of a concern for honesty and because I don't intend to be either hard-headed or hard-hearted. But henceforth I intend to address my readers' intelligence and no longer primarily their hearts.

Between the two is the need to lay down no absolutes and the need to show that human problems have everything to gain from rigorous intelligibility.

Interlude on Method

A society reveals itself by the way in which it treats certain significant phenomena. The problem of disability is one such phenomenon. To speak at all pertinently of disabled people is to disclose a society's depths. It amounts to saying that a book like this one, which is not divorced from praxis, is on a theoretical level from the very outset, on the level of the sociability (or sociableness; Fr. *sociabilité*) of a society, by which I mean its fundamental capacity to have people live together plus the anthropological information on that social competency.

Reassociating the question of the disabled with that of society presupposes substantial historical detachment. The matter is made even more difficult by the fact that historical works on this subject are uncommon and too selective.[11] But this presupposes, in addition, a question that has gone unnoticed, if we think that beyond the clichés there is still something to be discovered. It is common today to identify exclusion (at times quite subtle) and protest against it (an action always very divided). The reason for the exclusion can be pinpointed fairly easily: an economic system predicated on profitability; an economic system that can afford the luxury of generously helping its subjects, who are often its victims, but that considers prevention and sociovocational reintegration burdensome; a cultural system that no longer knows how to make difference viable because its schemas are those of identity, of "all the same"; a system of medical power based on the clinic and its history. We shall try here to ask the question in a different fashion: why does society try to integrate the disabled? What is behind this intention? And, more exactly, why does society want to integrate in the way that it does?

These questions can be asked of all societies, of all forms of sociopolitical organization. The question of integration seems even more general than that of exclusion, because—paradoxically, for our contemporary mentality—integration is more of a constant in human societies than exclusion. To initiate an analysis of the social workings of disability by way of its integration is a method more critical, even more militant, than to address it in terms of exclusion. The motives and factors that lead to rejection, even when such rejection is hidden and subtle, are fairly obvious to the attentive. Integration passes more unnoticed. Sometimes it even seems to occur on its own. It embodies claims that are widely supported today. Everything contributes to masking the reasons for integration, to forgetting them, to jumbling the various means of integration under the aegis of an ethics of integration. From the moment you integrate, who would venture

to come looking for how it happens, why it happens, and in the way
it does?

Today, for example, the endless goodwill of our liberals, often
enough similar to that of the Left, prevents us from questioning the
procedure itself. The most common slogan speaks of "being like the
others" (*être comme les autres*). A first line of inquiry comes to mind at
once: to be, or to seem to be, like the others? This is not a trifling
question. What is asked of people considered disabled? A secret, a lie,
a falsification? And why is this asked of them? And why may they
themselves demand it? Then there is the matter of being like the
others. Are they then all so similar, opposable as a group to a category
that may have no existence other than by the overly simple mechanism of a massive contrast? And who is supposed to be imitated in the
equation "like"? What kind of image is constructed socially of the
individual who is made the object of imitation? What is the cultural
model that is thus being imposed? To what society, to what type of
sociability, does this imitation refer?

The relevance of these questions about present intentions to integrate allows us, better than any other means, to investigate different
social environments. If efforts at integration are not a modern phenomenon and are a historical fact of other societies, it is possible to make
enlightening comparisons. A door opens on a history of disability. This
history appears all the more necessary in that our most current construction of our past, as of other cultures, suffers from being simplistic. In
fact, our prejudice of progress tends to make us look good. We were
preceded, we assume, by a kind of barbarity that excluded the disabled
or eliminated them. Inversely, we are haunted, in the face of certain
modern aberrations, by a kind of idealistic view of earlier societies or
other societies, which, not being industrialized, might have successfully realized integration. Before any effort at axiology, we do well to
undertake a differentiation of the forms of inclusion. The dilemma,
exclude or include, hides a whole series of exclusions that are not all the
same and of inclusions which are not commensurate. We could just as
well say that the dilemma is illusory. What are societies doing when
they exclude in one way or another and when they integrate in this
fashion or that? What do they say about themselves in so doing? The

study of everything that we could call the marginalized allows us to bring out previously ignored or neglected dimensions of that society. Even more: these are indicators of social and cultural dynamics.[12] That is, they testify not so much to where society is going as to the tensions that are resident in it. They do not constitute a model, but they may provide illumination. At a minimum (but in fact often achieving much more) they ask this question: what sort of person is acknowledged as normal in *each society?*

It is only at the cost of this research that we may have a serious hope of discriminating and of acquiring the means to effect choice. This observation, too, is part of this book. I would not want to evade the necessity of proposing social strategies. I would certainly subscribe to these lines by Foucault with regard to his study of the clinic:

> The research that I am undertaking here therefore involves a project that is deliberately both historical and critical, in that it is concerned—outside all prescriptive intent—with determining the conditions of possibility of medical experience in modern times. I should like to make it plain once and for all that this book has not been written in favor of one kind of medicine as against another kind of medicine, or against medicine and in favor of an absence of medicine. It is a structural study that sets out to disentangle the conditions of its history from the density of discourse, as do others of my works. (*The Birth of the Clinic* [New York: Random House, 1994], xix, trans. A. M. Sheridan Smith, from *Naissance de la clinique* [Paris: Presses Universitaires de la France, 1963], xv)

After distancing myself from any personal position, however, I will cover ground where Foucault chose not to go in his first works. I simply connect the two, history and its discourse, in a single work but distinguish very clearly within it my more contingent analysis and personal choices. Engaged professionally in the struggle to reduce the damaging effects of illness and of accident, I will not back off from the question of what to do. But I make claims for my analysis only for what it is: an analysis and not a set of prescriptions.

I have chosen a guiding question, and I aspire to a lucid inquiry. What will be the status of this undertaking?

A writer may dispense with displaying his methodology. Either he has an exact one and leaves to his readers the task of discovering it, or he has only partially developed it but judges his message more urgent and the epistemological preliminaries secondary. I shall not shy away from a few clarifying remarks on this matter.

Since I have a very high regard for science, I don't claim to aspire to it in this book. In brief, science's traditional route is approximately as follows: from an area of experiences one selects a phenomenon; from this is abstracted an object (the scientific object is always constructed), models are applied, purely formal if possible, and at a minimum interpretive. The impossibility of keeping to formal models—particularly in what are called the human sciences—is due to the recalcitrant nature of certain problems such as the single event or the unique. Thus, science most often ends up with typologies. A type is neither a class nor an individual; it is a "category of the structural kind," as G. G. Grangier says.[13] If we adhere to these characteristics of science, this undertaking concerning disability could not call itself science. Besides, since *Les Mots et les choses* of Foucault (1968), we know that the issue in the human sciences is neither to be science nor to speak of humanity but to draw the contours of the continent of alterity, for not only can the sciences "do without with the concept of humanity, they cannot penetrate it; they always address what constitutes its outer limits." These observations, which I am only just recalling here, are not aimed at making irrelevant the rigor that ought to inform a study even if it is not scientific in the accepted sense of the word. Nor do they claim that nothing is discovered of the human condition through all the explorations of the unconscious, of systems that are not manifest, of structures of meaning, and so on. Simply put, and this is the point that I want to stress, my intention is to exploit the rigor learned from the sciences—but engaged in human sciences it is not my ambition to establish a body of knowledge on disability and on the relationship between society and disability. At most my goal is to enlarge the understanding that we already have.

At the present time a historicist history of disability is not possible; there are too few in-depth studies. There are only soundings, as I earlier stated. On the other hand, on the basis of a learning that is as wide ranging as possible, one can engage in questions of a philosophical kind: what were the preconditions for differing social treatments of disability throughout history? When Foucault abandons the idea of writing a history of psychiatry—which would have risked valorizing the progress of therapy—it is in order to ask by which routes "madness" became "mental illness" and became the object of an appropriate medicine. The question is no longer strictly the historian's, and, if Foucault can be read as adducing elements for the historian (even fertile hypotheses),[14] he situates his intervention in the register of epistemology, now become archaeology, the very origin of the division between reason and unreason, and the construction of that division. Here, again, I shall limit myself to evoking from a distance the work of Foucault in order to situate the pages that follow. I will try to furnish extensive documentation, I will work with the greatest number of materials that my limitations permit, but I am guided by questions that go beyond a history of disability, that is, by questions that try to raise the veil on what is most hidden under this history. In so doing, it is certain that the history that one writes may to a great extent be fiction: "I am going to tell you the story of disability in a style and in a way that you wouldn't expect; now pay attention: once upon a time . . ." Two simple observations are called for: every history, even the historian's historicist history, is a *told* history. We cannot do otherwise, whatever guarantees we give—but, above all, when listening to my story, listen to the part that you have never heard before. And I do say *part* of this story of disability, for much as we must recognize the limits of the attempt, it would be equally foolish to denigrate the undertaking. Foucault, to take him once again as a reference point, has much to say on this subject, even—and especially—to the extent that one cannot know whether what one writes is objective. I hope to have much to say in the account I am about to construct, based as much as possible on documentation.

These documents differ greatly as concerns physical aberration. At times they belong to literature or to myth, at times to sociology. At times the inquiry must turn to medicine and at other times to economics. Here we are dealing with a history of mentalities and there with exact, incontestable events. We find social practices attested for one period, and for another we have scarcely more than commentary. Diverse and scattered, such is the state of our information. In addition, while trying to reconstitute the mental universes that governed the relationship between society and disability, I especially want to identify the distinctive features of cultures, even if these are very numerous. It is less an archaeology of knowledge that concerns me than a semiotics of cultures. That is, my interest is in the perception of cultural universes more than in the problems of knowing and doing. These emphases are not foreign to one another, but they do remain quite distinct.

In order that the reader remain well disposed, I must point out that this characterology of cultures, from the vantage point of disability, is only just sketched in. As testimony, I cite a very learned study on the role of disability in proverbs.[15] The author, by means of popular sayings, shows the variety of attitudes toward the disabled. Certainly, in these fixed patterns of thought constant features do appear, such as depreciation, the importance of blindness, the distinction between disabilities that lend themselves to begging and those that one hides (paralysis), but in the final analysis we cannot distinguish cultural eras. We find fear, rejection, exclusion, as well as the belief in special gifts of the disabled. Disabled people bring good luck and bad; they are beneficent or harmful. At the conclusion of this fascinating investigation, the author asks whether all this still shapes people's minds or whether proverbs refer only to the past, and he writes: "Only an intercultural study on the subject addressed here, a study which we wholeheartedly call for, would make an objective reply possible."

It is appeals of this kind that prompted me to deepen the anthropological aspect of this history, or, if you prefer, to give anthropology a historical dimension. In short, over the course of time I found myself deep into historical anthropology as André Burguière speaks of it, a subject without its own discipline but which "is equivalent to a procedure that always links the evolution under study to its social resonance, and to behaviors that it generated or modified,"[16] and again, when he says with great acuity: "The least discussed behavioral patterns of a society, like the care of the body, ways of dressing, the organization of work, and the calendar of daily activities reflect a system for the mental construction of the world that links them at the deepest level to the most developed of intellectual formulations, such as law, religious conceptions, philosophical or scientific thought" (159).

For the relationship between history and anthropology, it is appropriate to look back to the inaugural lecture of Claude Lévi-Strauss on his appointment to the chair of social anthropology:[17] "To scorn the historical dimension on the pretext that the means to evaluate it are insufficient in any but an approximate fashion leads to making do with a rarefied sociology in which phenomena are as if detached from their bases. Rules and institutions, states and processes seem to float in a vacuum in which the researcher strives to weave a subtle network of functional relationships. He becomes entirely absorbed in this task. And he forgets the human beings in whose thoughts these relationships were established, he neglects their concrete culture, he no longer knows where they come from nor who they are." These remarks are based on the reminder of Marcel Mauss: it is always a question of a given person or of a given society, of a given place, at a given moment. The originality of social anthropology, "instead of seeing causal explanation as the opposite of understanding, consists of discovering for oneself an object which is at the same time both very distant and subjectively very concrete, and whose causal explanation may be founded in that understanding which is for us only a supplementary form of proof" (17). We can interpret the very distant not only as that which affects societies quite different from our own, along the lines of classical anthropology, but also as the historical distance that we know must be put between ourselves and our objects of study. This is the more feasible, since in his text social anthropology is conceived of as a domain of the semiotics anticipated by Saussure; it sets out "the symbolic nature of its object of study." In fact, it is not because a fact can be called "social" that it belongs to the sphere of anthropology but because this social fact is significant "for anthropology, which is a person-to-person conversation; everything is a symbol and sign posed as intermediary between two subjects" (20). Social anthropology will always have as its "foundation a knowledge perfected in communication with its subjects."

The symbolic nature of the objects of anthropology also creates its necessary historicity. From the moment we raise structures and social processes to the status of signs, to be deployed as elements of an utterance, as a form of discourse, we cannot treat them otherwise than in their own situation, in context, which is also to periodicize and date them, make them singular: this is the work of history.

2

The Bible and Disability: The Cult of God

Exploring the situation of disability in Jewish culture and society up to the Christian era, we must admit that the social practices of this society are very difficult to determine. We have the text of the Bible. It is a prodigious document but, at the same time, one that conceals. We have only this text and parallel texts such as the Midrash or Talmudic writings. Recent years have witnessed the emergence of a reading, deceptively called materialist, that attempts to reconstitute the socio-political setting in which the biblical texts arose. But the extreme difficulty of such a reading is apparent, and the resulting hypotheses are still flimsy. It will then be evident that the present chapter is based only on the texts and not on a history of the Jewish society of the Old Testament.

Added to this constraint is the very taxing question of biblical hermeneutics, to use the phrase of exegetes. We have, first, a conflict in methods of textual analysis, which have been innumerable in the course of the history of theology and are still very diversified today after the appearance of psychoanalysis, Marxism, structuralism, and the multiple forms of semiotics. Second, as a consequence, we have a conflict in interpretation as concerns the meaning of the texts and their religious or philosophical implications. My reading—relying at times on semiotics, that is, the structural analysis of the text as text, will be guided by the basic question of this book: which representations and which *social* situations of disability are offered by these texts? What anthropological perspective supports the discourse of the biblical texts?

Prohibition

A considerable number of disabilities, if not all, both physical and mental, are mentioned in the Bible.[1] Disability was an everyday reality. But, as the text of Leviticus 21.16–24 reveals, it was also a sacred reality. Legal uncleanness was attached to the disabled, who could, of course, participate in cultic observances but never as priests who made sacrifices. The sanctuary could not be profaned. The disabled had the status of prostitutes or of women whom menstruation made unclean. One had to be without defect in order to approach God's place of residence.[2] Here we are faced with a *cultic* impurity.

The *Encyclopedia Judaica* develops this concept in the article "Blemish" by enumerating the impairments that preclude the offering of sacrifices: blindness and certain eye diseases,[3] injuries to the thigh,[4] a deformed nose (flattened between the eyes), lameness, the loss of a limb, skeletal deformation, muscle degeneration, a humped back,[5] skin diseases even if not precisely identified, the loss of a testicle. Yet the texts do distinguish among various deformities and illnesses. For example, the deaf and mute are subnormal according to Jewish law, while the blind are considered normal and enjoy their full rights. It has at times been said that the blind were looked on as persons who had died. The *Encyclopedia Judaica* sees this as only a rhetorical formula.[6] But all these distinctions in no way detract from the fundamental fact that disabilities as a whole were judged impurities, disqualifying their bearers from active participation in the cult.

In the Qumran texts, reflecting a late and admittedly Essene Judaism, we find an Essene regulation that denies the disabled engagement in combat on the one hand and participation in communal meals on the other. "And no man, lame, blind or crippled or having an incurable defect of the flesh, or afflicted by an impurity of the flesh, none of these shall accompany them to battle," and, in the appended regulation, "every person afflicted by these impurities, unsuited to occupy a place in the midst of the Congregation, and every person stricken in his flesh, paralyzed in the feet or hands, lame or blind or deaf or mute or stricken in his flesh with a defect visible to the eye . . . let not these persons enter to take a place among the Congregation of men of repute. And if one among them has something to say to the Council of Sanctity, he will be questioned apart; but this person shall not enter into the midst of the Congregation, for he is afflicted," and elsewhere "the slow-witted, the fools, the silly, the mad, the blind, the crippled, the lame, the deaf, the underage, none of these shall enter the bosom of the Community, for the holy angels dwell in its midst."[7]

The community of Qumran excluded the disabled of all kinds. This was a ritual exclusion, since it was in the name of the *sanctity* of the congregation or community that the exclusion was proclaimed. The ritual nature of the exclusion is confirmed by the Koran, which took up this Essene rule but adapted it:[8] the disabled are exempt from battle, not because of their uncleanness but simply because of their incapacity. And when the Prophet says, "No reproach to the blind, no reproach to the lame, no reproach to the sick," he wipes out the pollution of the disabled. He maintains the exemption from combat but completely removes the exclusion from meals. In this respect his position is identical to that of Jesus, who invited to his banquet "the crippled, the blind, the lame."[9] The Judaism of the Old Testament, on the other hand, is dominated by ritual, cultic prohibition, while the theological currents that derive from it (Christianity and Islam) differ on this point, as on others.

The Bible also reveals the social exclusion of certain illnesses. This is illustrated in a very long passage in Leviticus 13 and 14 dealing with leprosy. It may be summarized as follows: those whose skin is afflicted are examined by the priest, and, if the symptoms are found to be those of leprosy (or of a serious disease of the skin), he must deliver a judgment of "unclean." The priest functions here as a specialist who determines whether there is actually an impurity or not. This impurity entails a physical seclusion from the social group, which required, if a cure were to be sought, a purification ritual. The ritual was very precise and complex and permitted rehabilitation and reentry to ordinary life. The prohibition that weighs on the leper is legal, that is, provided for, codified, and not moral—but it is no less an exclusion from the group. As we see in Job 2.7–8, lepers were at times obliged to rites of mourning, which warned others to keep their distance from these unclean beings, excluded from the world of the living.

It is possible to link these prescriptions, first, to the draconian measures of cleanliness that are found in biblical tradition. It would then be a matter of a buffer zone to prevent contagion and protect the health of the group. It was all the more needed because physicians and medicine were ineffectual and not always highly esteemed. There is some humor at the expense of doctors and their limitations, even if at times they are honored (Pss. 38.1–15), instead of competing with the sole healer God (Exod. 15.26; 2 Kings 20.8).

This perspective amounts to bringing the prohibition down to a question of hygiene. But the link with the priesthood and with the sacred belies this single perspective. The impurity profanes the people. It should be recalled that the chapters of Leviticus that bracket those concerning leprosy deal with the purification of clean and unclean animals, of women after childbirth, and of sexual pollution. These different elements render unclean the places, objects, and persons with which they are in contact. The most current interpretation of this impurity refers it to a kind of taboo, which relieves anxiety in the face of the unknown, the uncommon, the altered. A defense is needed; the remedy lies in purification. It is evident that the social interdiction of certain kinds of disability reinforces the sacral interdiction with reference to religious practice: both bear witness to the foreignness of the affliction that must be averted and that cannot be referred back to God. In order to understand this social rejection of some illnesses (quite limited, we must insist), we must first grasp the implications of the sacral prohibition.

It is important to underline that in this fashion disability—of all sorts—is *situated*. It participates in the social division: in the opposition between sacred and profane, it is on the side of the profane. But disability is by no means alone there. It precludes participation in the priestly function, essentially understood as mediating between God and the people. But we should not neglect to note that for the Jewish people God is not everywhere; he is always present in the guise of *shekinah*, that is, very precise, very contingent: in the Ark of the Covenant, between the wings of the Seraphim, in the Temple and the Holy of Holies, and not elsewhere in the same capacity. This doubtless explains why instances that are excluded from this special point of encounter between the sacred and the profane still have to be dealt with socially. The sacred is quite limited, and God is too much an Other: instead, the sphere of the human, in particular the ethical sphere, is opened. This is evident under another aspect as well.

Defect is linked to sin—directly, for the Jewish religious conscience of the time. This is illustrated in the Pharisees' question to Jesus concerning a blind man: "Who sinned? Was it he or his family?" Is it wholly this tie between impairment and sin that drives the cultic interdiction? The defect linked to sin signifies that the affliction is to be associated with man and not with God. This is the Bible's basic statement on sin: man is the source of evil. It is not an inevitable destiny, nor is it an act of God. It is relatively simple to understand that this signification entails the pollution in disability: what derives from human sin has no part in God. But it is up to man to cure himself. Is it not because of this conception that a social morality is applied to disability? In the text of Exodus 21.28 ff. we meet the concept of reparation of the disability that has been caused. This idea of reparation can have far-reaching consequences, as the original text states: "When an ox gores a man or woman to death, the ox shall be stoned, and its flesh shall not be eaten; but the owner of the ox shall not be liable. If the ox has been accustomed to gore, and its owner has been warned but has not restrained it, and it kills a man or a woman, the ox shall be stoned, and its owner also shall be put to death. If a ransom is imposed on the owner, then the owner shall pay whatever is imposed for the redemption of the victim's life. If it gores a boy or girl, the owner shall be put to death according to the same rule. If the ox gores a male or female slave, the owner shall pay to the slave owner thirty shekels of silver, and the ox shall be stoned" (Exod. 21.28–32).

Here we have a whole legislation and jurisprudence for indirect liability, social liability. A comparison with present-day workplace accidents springs spontaneously to mind! But rather than comment on this form of elevated retributive justice, I would insist on the consistency of Jewish thought. Sin and defect deny the disabled a religious role, but they introduce an ethical and social imperative. The person who is so tried is not condemned, even if the religious signification that he bears dooms him to a very precise and circumscribed form of exclusion.

Moreover, awareness of this condition can only be heightened when, as in Job's case, physical (and social!) ills are quite divorced from any direct connection with personal sin. Job sees all sorts of disasters befall him but proclaims his innocence. This surplus of misfortune is not, however, attributed to Him, who remains the Other. It is then a fact to be dealt with on the human level but one that still does not overwhelm the person who is its victim. Job paves the way for the critical responsibility of human beings for one another. We are mutually accountable for our fellows.

The celebrated texts of the prophecy of Isaiah, currently called the Songs of the Suffering Servant,[10] make of this servant—who is difficult to identify: is it the people of Israel, is it a group, is it an individual?—the distillate and representative of suffering, who bears all the sin of the human collectivity. He, too, is innocent. He, too, bears witness to the innocence of God. But he, too, refers back to the conduct of people one to another. It is reciprocal violence among men, social violence, that is highlighted, denounced, and summoned to conversion.

Before examining the coherence of the Jewish system, it seems useful to seek out the cornerstone of this social construction of Israel. At the very moment when the name Israel is accorded to the Hebrew people, the subject of disability arises. Let us read the biblical text, much older than those that deal with interdictions, in which it tells of someone who becomes disabled—the celebrated account of the nocturnal combat of Jacob, a combat that leaves him lame (Gen. 32.23–33). Of course, it is not possible to associate this text directly with the social problem of the impaired. Jacob's lameness, subsequent to his struggle, is the mark of a very special situation. Yet the signification of this affliction may illuminate biblical mentality as concerns disability. Let us examine just how, by unraveling the weave of the text.

Jacob, who has remained alone, wrestles long through the night with an anonymous being who dislocates his hip. He is victorious, and his adversary seeks to flee, but Jacob imposes a contract: he must bless Jacob in return for his release. Jacob receives a new name, while his opponent remains nameless. Jacob interprets this polemical and adversarial encounter as a vision of God, however, and he rejoices at coming from the combat alive. But he comes away injured, just as he comes away newly named. His disability is a mark, a mark of difference. Everything in the text combines to signify this alterity: night, anonymity, the defeated contestant who still has the power to name; a whole series of oppositions are at play in the text (high/low, dusk/dawn). Lameness is the double sanction for the difference confronted and for belonging to the earth, to the human condition, while the new name and the blessing bring him out of his former condition. Undergoing the test against the Other, Jacob is himself altered, but he remains more than ever earthbound. He is the conquering hero who achieves the object of his desire but who is recalled to his terrestrial affiliation. His disability separates him from the zone interpreted as divine. His virile strength is diminished, and this affliction leaves him a stranger to God. It is less the mark of God on him than the mark that he will not partake fully of God. For, if the new name and the blessing are euphoric sanctions, lameness is dysphoric. It signifies that he did not dominate his adversary, whom he nonetheless held off. He is not of the same order as his opponent. Disability is the uncommon element, but this uncommonness establishes the difference between the Other and earthly man. It is then given certain implications in the religious relationship; it constitutes a kind of dividing line. One does not cross over the boundary of the sacred. Before any explicit interdiction arises to inscribe this conception in law and social order, disability serves to separate what is God's from what is man's, the sacred from the profane. The account of Jacob at the ford of Jabbok testifies to the essentially religious context in which disability is situated in the Bible.

The System

Before exploring the system of thought that permits the double practice of religious prohibition and ethical obligation in early Judaism, it is important to examine the denunciation of violence done to the unfortunate and disfigured.

Here it is worthwhile to recall the analysis of René Girard.[11] For this author understanding human relations, social relations, requires that we first address violence. In fact, human desire is mimetic; it seeks to appropriate the desire and the objects of desire of another. The crisis that is the consequence can be resolved only by the ritual sacrifice of a victim, a scapegoat that makes it possible to expel the violence and to leave the possibility of a livable common space. This victim mechanism not only deflects violence (although always only temporarily) but also conceals it. The group forgets that it is founded on the sacrifice of victims, sacralized outlets, and that sacrifice entails radical violence. Girard attempts to explain the totality of ethnological and anthropological data (including our complex societies) on the basis of this fundamental phenomenon. Among other things, he shows how all prohibitions are connected to it. These serve to prevent a generalized mimesis; that is, they curb desire and prevent it from developing into such rivalry that absolute violence would break out and jeopardize society itself. It does seem that the biblical text exposes a very profound violence, as concerns disability and physical and mental ills. The person who is afflicted is made to bear the burden of sin, the burden of wrongdoing. We are not very far from the phenomenon of the scapegoat. Ritual interdiction is one form of it. But at the same time we are in the presence of a radical social responsibility for evil, and thus for misfortune. As a consequence, and from another perspective, the religious prohibition that weighs on the disabled, that is, their distancing from the presence of God, allows social responsibility to come into play. Two opposing tendencies seem to me to run through the Judaism of the Old Testament: that of violence, sacral order, and religious order, which tends to make the disabled one of the expelled victims, and that of ethics and social order, which strives not to contaminate the divine and, in contrast, to assume the obligation to situate the disabled within society.

In support of this conception, let us engage in some theological reasoning. If the disabled were related to the divine, God would have a part in them and would not be foreign to them. Society would be, to some degree, relieved of responsibility. But then why could the deformed person not serve as a victim? From an exclusively religious standpoint it is almost logical to proceed with the sacrifice of abnormal beings. Old Testament Judaism does not do this, because its religion is not simply composed of sacral logic but also of ethical logic. And this is doubtless due to the very notion of God that it formed: God is entirely Other (there is no image of him). If he is then Other, he could not have any relationship with us in which mimesis played a role. God and man do not imitate each other. Their difference cannot be resolved in any fashion. Nor is abnormality, which obviously cannot signify God's difference because of the interdiction, of any value in a sacrifice, since sin is our fault alone. God is totally foreign to our violence, and, as a result, he refers us back wholly to our own responsibility. The aberrant, by being religiously unclean, is no more suitable for sacrifice than for sacralization. In other words, and here I return to one of the ideas of Girard, biblical Judaism, although still containing a sacrificial mechanism, begins to perceive that the poor, the crippled, the abnormal, are *innocent,* that they are not to be exploited as scapegoats.

These, then, are the contours of the very strong coherence of the ancient Jewish system. A religious prohibition without possibility of appeal affects all the categories of what we group under the term *disabled.* A religious prohibition linked to a certain representation of God that explains that the interdiction itself exonerates the impaired and refers the problem back to an ethics of social responsibility. We could say, almost without paradox, that the nonintegration of the disabled in religious practice is the precondition of their nonexclusion from the culture.

Just how is this possible? In this biblical culture two levels of thought dominate and intersect. The first level, or what we might better call the first isotopy,[12] is religious. This register, very pregnant with meaning and dominant in all societies of antiquity, has as its prime function to separate divine order from profane order—but at the very same time, and just as important, to establish the distinction between nature and culture. Its third function is to define, on a more ethical level, what is natural and what is aberrant. This religious isotopy meets a biological isotopy: there are healthy bodies and others that are sick, well-formed bodies and deformed bodies, there is the normal and the monstrous, the natural and the aberrant.

The religious level, if left to itself, would supply the principle of exclusion for that which was abnormal on the biological level. The religious level is *also ethical;* it is ethical and religious at the same time. The categories of this ethical-religious plane are pluralistic, since they derive from a complex isotopy composed of two sub-isotopies. We may superpose the following oppositions: sacred/profane, which the religious prohibition emphasizes so strongly; divine/malign, for impurity is not divorced from sin (collective wrongdoing long before it became individual); fortune/misfortune, because the disabled and poor, even though objects of pity, compassion, are no less to be counted among the suffering.

Thus, one could represent the basic organization of the biblical system in the form of a simple graphic. All outlines are reductive, but they facilitate the debate of essentials.

Biological level (or isotopy)

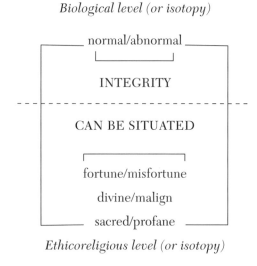

Ethicoreligious level (or isotopy)

This system is that of *the integral* and *the situable.* In fact, the opposition between normal and abnormal produces an idea of integrity as a natural element. What is natural is integral. This may seem banal, because this division of things is so often to be found. But, as I shall demonstrate, this is no longer true in our society, where the natural is not primarily the condition of being *integral* but that of being *integrable.* This will become the new social naturalness. It is no less true that what a society calls natural is a relative cultural datum. But this idea of integrity, which the Bible shares with many other early societies, is *situated* on the ethical-religious level. Nonintegrity creates a distance from a precise religious function, but this same function, because of the notion of God that it implies, obliges us to a moral view of the aberrant.

Breakdown of the Prohibition?

Up to this point our thesis has been that the situation of the disabled in the Israel of the Old Testament was shaped by religious prohibition and that, even if there were an aspect of social rejection, in certain quite specific cases, by reason of fear and for prophylaxis, there was a social integration thanks to an elevated ethic directed by the very presence of the interdiction.

Was this coherence not undone when the great disrupter of Jewish religion called Jesus of Nazareth appeared? He encountered many sick and crippled people. This is, moreover, one of the factors that give the Gospels so much of their tenderness. Without denying the global connection between evil (and misfortune) and sin, Jesus quite decisively breaks the connection between disability and individual fault. But, otherwise, he does not seem to allude to the justification of the religious prohibition that affects the impaired. The practice of Jesus the Nazarene is relief and cure. It is certainly true that, in a contemporary reading of the New Testament, the cures have a signification that goes beyond the miraculous. It could even be claimed that it is scarcely ever a question of a miracle in the current sense of the term. Healing partakes of a textual economy, the analyses of which are, moreover, multiple. We are not engaged here in exegesis nor in theology; these are not our debates. But it is claimed that Jesus had to have known disability. In going out to those who were under the interdiction (lepers, the blind, prostitutes, etc.) or in letting them come to him, he was performing less a social act than an act to deconstruct the religious mentality. To me Jesus seems to be the wrecker of the prohibition. But this is fraught with consequences, for the whole Jewish system was erected on it. The reverse side of interdiction was a certain integration. Exploding the prohibition makes necessary the creation of a new social system as well. Society has been destabilized.

Jesus says explicitly that the sick, the disabled, the marginalized, are the first in the Kingdom of God. His affection for them is due to their closeness to God; he cites them as examples of faith and of grace. To be sure, he does at times send them back to the priests for a rite of purification; it is equally true that it is when *healed* that some of them become his disciples or his proselytizers. But it is no less true that he suspends the ancestral prohibition. Indirectly at first. Each time there is a question of clean and unclean (alimentary prohibitions, Mark 7.19 ff.; daily ritual prescriptions, Matt. 15.11; Jewish-pagan relations, Acts 10.28, etc.),[13] the New Testament text subverts the traditional conception. The wrong does not lie in exterior pollution; it lies in the conduct of one person toward another. It is what a person says or does to his fellow that constitutes uncleanness. Purity and impurity are in the relations that one maintains or establishes. Man's heart is answerable for all, as the text says.

This is extremely important. While before the coming of Jesus the pure and impure comprised two objective zones, after and because of him it is human beings who create and demarcate them. Under the Old Covenant impurity afflicted the disabled, and, as a consequence, requirements and restrictions were generated. Under the New Covenant all responsibility devolved on mankind. In other words, ethics became primary. It is not simply a consequence of sacral arrangements; it becomes their basis. There is no distinction of sacred and profane. Only one thing is sacred, and that is human fellowship, which can be profaned by lack of respect, lack of love, lack of *agape.* The question is no longer whether you are purified but whether you have a pure heart. In a formulation that is no doubt incomplete we could state that Jesus causes the religious element to cede in favor of the ethical. Or, rather, he changes the conception of the religious from top to bottom. The religious is first of all the bond among human beings, as it is first of all the love that unites God to man. When these ties are of love, the religious, thus the sacred, thus the pure, are present; when these ties are degraded, the impure arises, the profane enters, the religious is effaced. The old divisions are muddled, and new divisions appear. This quite remarkable aspect of the Gospels has not been sufficiently noted: there is no other sacred than the relations to one's fellows. The sacred, conceived as affecting places, times, things, or functions, and dismissing the rest to the zone of the profane, no longer exists. The only sacred thing is man and woman.

But it is not simply in indirect fashion that Jesus raised the prohibition that concerns us here. The Sabbath corresponded in time to the Temple in space: the place reserved for God where all kinds of things are forbidden, including the care and healing of the sick. And it is on the Sabbath that we see Jesus cure a blind man, in chapter 9 of the well-known text of John.[14] And this is one of the arguments of the Pharisees, those inflexible censors but faithful guardians of legality, to have Jesus declared a sinner and to convince the disabled old man to see the work of the devil in his cure. The most fundamental categories are called back into question. If we see little of Jesus in contact with the disabled in the Temple (while he meets them several times in the synagogue, which is not a sacred place of residence of God), it is simply because the prohibition was in full force. The subversion of the Sabbath should be understood equally well as the subversion of the Temple. One text even bears witness to this subversion of the Temple: in Matthew 21.24 the blind and the lame approach Jesus in the Temple, and Jesus heals them. As we have seen, the blind and lame headed the list of those excluded from the Temple (2 Sam. 5.8).

But in shattering the prohibition, the texts of the Gospels put the integration of the unfortunate back into the hands of ethical and spiritual conscience. The interdiction excluded in well-defined terms, but it also protected the impaired. Now there is no longer exclusion, but the impaired are even more exposed. The legal violence done to the poor is denounced, but society is even more returned to its violence, of which it can be quit only through love. With the Gospels a completely different system begins for the disabled. Their dignity, their right to partake fully of religious and social life, are recognized. But is misfortune any the more averted? It can no longer be warded off in the same way. A completely new form of integration—and of exclusion—

has been introduced. In what follows it will be the sole principle of charity that we shall be dealing with: charity that must be understood here in its root sense, not in its commonplace sense, but in the sense of *agape,* disinterested love composed of goodwill and respect for equality, well summarized in the word *fellowship.* Will the Gospel principle find a social path? What will be the hazards, for the culture, in this vision? What kinds of prohibitions will reappear? The former coherence has been destroyed, a new coherence is proposed, but it is entirely and solely dependent on responsibility. How will conscience and the practices of the Christian society to be established in the West adapt the new perspective?

Whether, as in Jewish tradition, we do not consider the two bodies of texts commonly called biblical (i.e., the Old and New Testaments) to be linked or whether, on the contrary and as in the Christian tradition, we take them as books of equal and interdependent importance, the break between the Jewish Bible and the Gospel seems to me to be irresolvable. The New Testament text undermines one of the two pillars on which the earlier system was constructed. First, there is ethics.[15] Moreover, the rigor of the new logic must be emphasized, as must that of its predecessor. In fact, the God of the New Testament is above all a God-relationship: a relationship within himself (Father, Son, Holy Ghost), relationship with mankind (he proposes a covenant in the very person of Jesus). The God-relationship no longer entails religious prohibitions, just the opposite; it excludes only the wicked heart, only the wrong that comes from within. But, then, at the same time, and this has hardly been emphasized either, we find ourselves facing a problem that is extremely difficult to assume: our relationship to disability, our relationship to abnormality, depends entirely on ourselves. There are no longer any dictates; there is nothing preestablished that would permit a social order. The Gospels disturb, deconstruct, sow panic, and become a source of instability. The principle of charity alone and no longer the prohibition reveals a problem that the Christian tradition has never resolved, one for which it remains in continuous debate and in awesome ineffectiveness: how can charity be the organizing principle of a society? This problem, which is so vast and which could summarily represent a very considerable part of Christian history, will be pursued from the vantage point of this question: how will charity seek to be a principle for organizing aberrancy? Many subsystems will be tested and our own in the twentieth century is still partially derivative of the break that was introduced by the texts of the Gospels.

3

Western Antiquity:
The Fear of the Gods

Praxis

Deformity Put Aside, Weakness under Care

The West draws on two sources: Judaism and classical antiquity. It is not my purpose to distinguish their relative shares of influence, even if that were possible. But to what extent does the Jewish system based on the Bible that was outlined in chapter 2 resemble or differ from Greco-Roman antiquity?

If we are to believe Marie Delcourt,[1] the practice established for *deformed infants* consisted of exposure, in Athens as well as in Sparta, and in early Rome. This applied only to deformities that were close to monstrosity, the *terata*. But malformations that are benign in our eyes, such as clubfoot, webbed hands, fused fingers, supernumerary digits, were considered deformities. What counts is the aberrant character in relation to the species and not the medical or adaptive seriousness of the abnormality. As soon as we face a birth that lacks the integrity recognized for the human race, we are in the sphere of *teratology*. This is sharply distinct from debility or illness. The conception of disability is very precise and does not cover the entire field of what today goes under this term.

The exposure of deformed infants means taking them outside the settlement to an unknown location and letting them expire in a hole in the ground or drown in a course of water. If the consequence is indeed death, the signification of exposure is not as an execution of these infants. Exposing them is only returning them to the gods. They are not killed; they are sacrificed to the gods. Although there is an expiatory character to this praxis, it cannot be referred to ritual sacrifice.[2] But there is a very pronounced religious sense in this: these births signal the possibility of misfortunes and are explained by the anger of the gods. Deformed infants are exposed because they are *harmful, maleficent.* They implicate the group. This is why they are exposed only by the decision of a council of wise men; it is not usually the parents who are in charge of such a matter, but the social body, the state.[3] In the case of Sparta, Delcourt writes: "If they were exposed, it is because they caused fear: they were the sign of the gods' anger and they were also the reason for it. This is symptomized by a concomitance where the untrained mind distinguishes poorly between cause and effect" (39). Precautions have to be taken, this is the essential concept, for "the preeminent sign sent by the gods to guilty men is the abnormal newborn, a sign that always arouses anxiety" (47).

Only much later does there appear a rationalization that justifies exposure on the grounds of eugenics or the impossibility of mixing good blood with bad.[4] At the root of this is a religious phobia, at times associated with sterility or in any case of the same order: the divine curse. Abnormal births are *expiated,* by public order. Monstrosities are linked to the fear of collective sterility, to a fear of the extinction of the species or of its departure from the norm. But this possible insecurity is not only biological, it is insecurity in face of the divine, linked to the wrongdoing of men and anger from above. This is why the act is not primarily a killing but a return to the hands of the gods. In this, the biological abnormality—for it is indeed an abnormality of the body, identified and designated—is projected onto the social level. In other words, aberrancy within the species not only threatens the future and the continuation of this species, but also announces, threatens, signifies a condemnation by the gods: a condemnation of the group. The biological and social levels are mingled, or rather create an isomorphism: an aberrancy within the corporeal order is an aberrancy in the social order (as in the moral order). This cannot be a private matter; it is not a medical matter. Nor is it a question for psychology. The differing body is socialized.[5]

Here it is exclusively a question of differing bodies, and not of weakened bodies. Antiquity quite clearly distinguished among malformation, mental retardation, and illness. Atonement through exposure is relevant only to that which threatens the norms of the human social species and not to a simple diminution, which can be accommodated. Thus the blind, the deaf, and the feeble-minded are not categorized among the deformed.[6] Cicero will later say to what extent blindness and deafness can be rewarding special characteristics. It is possible not only to compensate for them, but there are also "pleasures of the dark and of silence" that cannot be enjoyed by those who see and hear.[7] This demonstrates, in any case, that in antiquity sensory disruption was not connected with physical malformation. It might be congenital or adventitious but did not signify deviance within the species. It did not jeopardize conformity, did not point to a curse. Sensory disruption was a weakness, an illness.

To be sure, the distinction between malformation and deficiency is not always perfectly clear. Aulus Gellius, toward the end of the classical period, bears witness to this vacillation. He begins, however, with an opposition between *illness,* in which he includes, for example, both consumption and blindness, and *defect,* where he classifies stuttering along with malformation. He questions whether one should make distinctions based on the definitive or on the transitory nature of the affliction. He cites a civil law tract in which the madman and the mute are designated "ill," thus blurring the categories.[8] But this text, even if it testifies to some indecision, also establishes the difference between deficiency and defect. It would seem that for Greco-Roman antiquity the most acute problem was congenital malformation, the sole source of religious terror and the reason for fatal exclusion.

The practice of exposure, as distinct from statements on deficiency, is indicative of the classification of disabilities—and, moreover, of the mental universe underlying these divisions—in Western antiquity. Medical literature confirms these cultural data. Although I have chosen to begin by commenting on classical antiquity without going farther back in time, it is of some interest to look briefly elsewhere.[9] In Mesopotamian culture illness—and physical malformation as well—are linked to sin, to wrongdoing, which has its seat in human beings: adultery, incest, pollution. An individual may have committed a sin unknowingly. The sick person has been rejected by God and, in certain cases, should be rejected by the human community. Diseases come from the gods as a punishment,[10] or at least as a sign of their disapproval. As a consequence, recovery consisted in the first hand of seeking out the original wrong, even back through several generations, because a sick person could atone for earlier wrongdoing. The medicine that derives from this conception is psycho-moral in nature, not organic.

To continue with Marcel Sendrail, the mental universe changes completely among the Egyptians. Here we confront a magical universe. It is no longer an instance of punishment for sin but of metaphysical drama. Far beyond our human conduct there is the hostility of uncontrollable forces. Behind our transgressions, there is a rupture, both cosmic and divine. Misfortune and suffering are only the consequences of a previous breakdown. In this philosophical environment, illness and disability are better distinguished, while in Babylon and Sumer, everything was mixed together in expiation for sin. Here, in the valley of the Nile, which has left us important iconographical testimony on physical deformation, certain disabled persons play a social role. We see dwarves receiving honors or being carried on altars. The disabilities are not primarily pathogenic; the pathology of disease is consigned to a rite, to charms, in short, to something shamanistic.

This is a natural consequence of the more metaphysical than ethical mode of representation in ancient Egypt. It is less a question of atonement than of deflection, less inquiry than conciliation. "The punishment of a sin, known or unknown, for the Babylonians, the transposition to the human scale of a cosmic drama for the Egyptians, disease becomes both trial and sacrifice for the Hebrews. Moral disorder among the first-named, magical phenomenon among the second, display of the sacred among the third" (73). In what camp were the Greeks?

Before, and also coincidentally with, the appearance of more rational, technical, even clinical thought that is associated with Hippocrates, Greece was permeated by a current of the tragic. Above all, it was a matter of destiny. Beside a medicine where the objectives and the exercise of empirical knowledge were dawning, Greek thought saw in disease a sign of the ill will of the gods. This opposition between the Greek medicine of Hippocrates and the tragic is not absolute. The Greek world is more ambiguous, more mixed. Hellenic rationality does not stand opposite the irrationality of life. Not only is it a rationality that has been won from perception of the disorder and ruses of the world, it is a rationality always crossed by the tragic. Greek thought is a mixture of the tragic and the rational. Even if Plato is not always most representative of the common mentality, he illustrates the ambivalent status of illness when he proposes an itinerary of purification, from the logic of a perspective in which the soul is superior to the body, and matter is under the control of the spirit.

It should be noted, however, that in the two currents, Hippocratic and tragic, a common idea is formulated: we are under the regimen of necessity (*anankè*), under the control of the Nature of things. Even if there is a physical purification to be carried out, disease is chiefly to be referred to this natural order, either to point up the gap between the two or to signify the Necessity from which even the gods themselves cannot escape. The first hypothesis—disease as natural disorder—opens the way to empirical, scientific research on physical and biological rationality that has been disrupted. We witness the birth of Hippocratic medicine and the appearance of what will be the main stream of Western medicine. The second hypothesis—disease as a superior destiny—brings us back to physical deviance. We are dealing with a different order, that of the gods or at least one in which the gods are more proximate. *Disorder,* as represented by a certain number of morbidities, refers to a menace that actually belongs to a different order.

Thus, I believe that Delcourt was right when she claimed that exposure is a means of returning to the gods. At the same time, it is evident that on the basis of a collective cultural idea of necessity and thus of a notion of *order,* the division set out earlier remains valid: the Greek world makes a clear distinction between illness as weakness and illness as defect, although some words such as *nosos* have both meanings. These first illnesses belong to the sphere of technical medicine, the second to philosophical and social reflection. Delcourt somewhat overemphasizes, perhaps, the *human* fault that could be confused with individual fault. The sign of misfortune, of the divine curse, if you will.

Expiation up to a certain point, that is, submission to an Order that is unknown, terrifying, other, but not a sacrifice for a fault that has been *committed*, in the same sense as in Babylon. At the heart of the matter is the tragic flaw. And is not the tragic precisely the conflict between orders? Indeed, some pathologies make us fear for our own order—and society defends itself against them. But do they not refer, in terms of priority, to an order that threatens to crush our own?

Before entering this debate, the privileged venue of which will be the mythological corpus, it will be rewarding, by way of counterpoint, to examine aberrations that run parallel to those which interest us here.

What was the status of mental retardation, of mental affliction, of "madness"? In *The Laws*[11] Plato says that "the insane should not appear in the city, but each of them shall be kept in the home by those close to him." Then Plato gives as a reason for this recommendation the disruption, aggression, and danger that the madman provokes by his threatening or obscene words. And we know that in Athens the mentally ill were shunned: people threw stones at them or spit on them.[12] Besides terror, the insane also inspired respect everywhere, for common belief, drawing on very ancient ideas, saw in madness the intervention of the supernatural. Mental disorder is synonymous with possession, in the literal sense of the word.

On this basis Plato elaborated a conception of insanity that he called prophetic, in addition to ritual madness, poetic madness, and erotic madness.[13] These forms of insanity, especially the prophetic one, which is at work in oracles, for example, are very clearly distinguished from common madness. "When grievous maladies and afflictions have beset certain families by reason of some ancient sin, madness has appeared among them, and breaking out into prophecy has secured relief by finding the means thereto, namely by recourse to prayer and worship, and in consequence thereof rites and means of purification were established" (Plato, *Phaedrus,* 22).

Ordinary madness is associated with some wrongdoing for which compensation must be paid. The inspired, prophetic madmen break this cycle. I will not detail Plato's full thought on such delirium, which has a philosophical and purgative function; it reveals a science and an intention under the appearance of chaos (Dodds, *Les Grecs et l'irrationnel*, 82). Conventional insanity does not have this scope.[14] In both cases, as in that of physical aberrancy, we are dealing with the divine, even supra-divine, order. But the madman is not exposed; he is simply avoided. Why this difference? Doubtless because it is possible, if we follow Plato's thought, to integrate madness into a kind of revelation: it is one more means of access. Moreover, it can be warded off by the superior forms of madness. Physical aberrancy is crude, without a way out, in the final analysis more threatening. Without anticipating remarks to come, I should call attention to the obvious contrast with present-day culture, which maintains a much more problematic relationship with mental disorder than with physical deformity. This is because the relationship of reason/unreason, rational/irrational is not the same. The Greeks, although avid for the intelligible and for intellectual clarity, did not fail to recognize the supernatural interference on the one hand, the seductive obscurity of unreason on the other.[15]

The attitude toward congenital deformity and that toward insanity are not the only areas in which antiquity speaks to us of disability. We encounter many well-known malformations: club feet, Pott's disease, atrophy, poliomyelitis, etc. We see physicians attending to all the traditional illnesses: dermatosis, tuberculosis, nephritis, hepatitis, and so on, even though blindness and certain epidemics are of major concern. We also meet those wounded in war and the victims of accidents: "if the large Greek cities had state-paid physicians to care for the wounded without charge from the time of the wars against the Medes, the smaller cities were also prepared to make substantial sacrifices for the relief of their war wounded."[16] All kinds of inscriptions, stelae, and scattered texts attest to the existence of military medicine and, thus, of wounded veterans who were taken under public care. With a degree of randomness that we need not explore at present. We can see from a plea by Lysias, "For the Cripple" (from between 400 and 360 B.C.E.),[17] that disabled people of few means were to receive a pension determined annually by the Council of Athens. Candidates for this subsidy appeared before the Council, which reviewed their claim on the public purse, passed judgment, and supported or rejected the claim. Lysias is defending a disabled small merchant who found his right to a pension challenged by another citizen. This text is not very far-ranging, but it does witness to public aid instituted on behalf of citizens who were denied a living by disability, and to the allocation of appropriate public resources. Lysias clears his client of the various indictments: yes, he is misshapen, you have only to look; he can ride a horse, but the horse is borrowed; he is without extensive resources, because he is not of the well-to-do stratum of citizens. But this text does not tell us what the disability was, no more than it gives information on the general social condition of the impaired. The only thing that this speech confirms for us is that the city concerned itself with making available a minimum of resources to its impaired and impoverished veterans, in the form of an annual grant that might or might not be renewed. This was the situation in the Greek cities of the classical period.

This is, however, indicative of the classification of the impaired. On one side, congenital deformity is exposed; on another, mental illness is hidden but is not a cause for exclusion, with the possibility that it may bear a message for our world; on a third side, illness and adventitious disability are treated and cared for. We are very far from the kinds of classification that will later be made, and from those of the present day in particular. To avoid giving the impression that this classification is too rigid, it should be noted that physical disability, such as blindness, may also be the medium of a message. Tiresias is a seer.

Up to this point I have been concerned with what social praxis tells us on the one hand, and with the conception of illness on the other. But the most important topic remains to be explored: this society's discourse on the subject of aberrancy. I believe, in fact, that whatever its effective, empirical conduct, a society reveals just as much about itself by the way it speaks of a phenomenon. The imaginings of society—social imagination in its broadest sense—are a constituent of a society just as much as its praxis. We must break the habit of referring everything back to praxis. The gap between praxis and the collective "imaginary" may be large, and be due to quite other reasons than ideology in the Marxist sense of the word. The social imagination is also social reality.

The Myths

In order not to get off course in an overly long discussion of the definition of myth, I shall use this term for the literary corpus on which the classical mentality drew as a common source. This will include the *Iliad*, the *Odyssey*, as well as a large portion of Greek theater. This universe gives rise to certain very characteristic myths, such as that of Oedipus extended by Sophocles into the truly tragic. As we shall see, I give preferential status to Sophocles' version, because it occupies a more important place than others in discussions about Greece.

The accounts and stories of the gods are populated by disabilities that are there to play a structural role (and a structuralist one as well), and not as simple folkloristic details. The principals here are Oedipus and a number of figures close to him, the god Hephaestus, Philoctetes, even Hermaphrodite, to name only the major ones. The fundamental discourse of the Greeks and other ancient peoples includes malformation and anomalies. It would be very surprising if they were present for no other reason than as ornamentation.

Oedipus: The Operation of Difference
The myth of Oedipus is without qualification one of the major founding myths in antiquity as well as in the West; from Sophocles to Freud and Lévi-Strauss it has not ceased to be taken up again, reinterpreted and reworked.[18] And here, at the very outset of this myth, so essential to our culture and the inspiration of so much symbolism, is situated the problem of disability: Oedipus, variously lame, with swollen or pierced feet, is an exposed infant.[19] Is it because of his disability? Or is his disability adventitious, the result of his unlucky birth, due, for example, to the crime of homosexual rape committed by an ancestor? In actual fact, in ancient Greece exposure was not always motivated by deformity. If the disability of Oedipus could legitimately be seen to play the principal role in his exposure and thus in his fate, then one of the heroes most charged with significance would carry the stigmata of deficiency as a basic constituent and not as an accessory. Such a statement may appear shocking, but may it not be for reasons other than

the elements of the myth that we hesitate to entertain just this reading among others? What causes horror and fear, is it not that the otherness, even the monstrousness, should be *original*? The legend of Oedipus itself reveals this dread. It is true that people will not permit their heroes—even the tragic ones—to be the bearers of defects. At least, this is how Delcourt accounts for the transfer of the defect burdening the grandson to the grandfather (Labdabos, the lame),[20] since for her there is a transfer, even though a whole race or line of descent (*genos* in Greek) is involved, that is the object of divine condemnation and that is implicated in the problem of power. We find here again the characteristic ambiguity of the Greeks. Into the heart of the myth itself, a game of hide-and-seek has been introduced, one that shows the impossibility of separating opposed elements, contrary desires, irreconcilable thoughts.

That disability, aberration, anomaly and abnormality, malformation—like the affective relationship with kin, the relationship with the gods, the relationship to truth—are part of the fundamental problems of the human condition and of our culture is a conception perhaps not foreign to Greek thought. Claude Lévi-Strauss sees this clearly since he makes physical disability one of the four oppositional elements that structure myth.[21] We know that Lévi-Strauss identifies four columns, opposed two by two, in which all the components of myth are situated: one column where he inscribes all the "overvalued" kinship relations, another where all the "undervalued" kinship relations are located. These two columns constitute the first opposition. Then follow two other series: elements that mark a passage beyond the human condition and disabilities that recall the earthly tie: the second opposition. The two major oppositions themselves correspond to one another and can be expressed in the form of an equation.

Lévi-Strauss interprets this double opposition as a statement of the general problem of the same and the other. There is the superhuman and the ordinarily human, just as there is the incestuous relationship (identity, identicalness) and the relationship to the woman who is not the mother (alterity). In the same fashion, starting with the question of incest and the superhuman, there is the problem of our origin: are we born of two different beings or of one? The myth of Oedipus constitutes an accumulation of oppositions, each of which refers to a principal interrogation of humanity, and all of which refer one to another. Vast combinatorics, prodigious play of mirrors.

In the analysis of Lévi-Strauss physical malformation signifies two things. It is interpreted as the notice of our terrestrial affiliation, heavy and entangling. But it also enters into the opposition between terrestrial and divine, itself interpreted as posing the following question: do humanity's origins lie with the divine, and thus with that which is identical to itself, or with the earth, site of diversity and multiplicity?

Does recognizing with Lévi-Strauss that disability occupies a major place in the myth of Oedipus oblige us to follow him in his reading of the myth and in the methodology that he employs? In this account, is Oedipus a deformed infant and exposed because of it? Delcourt's elucidation, infinitely cautious, still seems convincing to me. At the outset of her book she states: "In an earlier book I tried to show that Oedipus is one of the unlucky newborns that ancient communities rid themselves of because their deformity was proof of divine anger."[22] To highlight the special case of Oedipus, the author reviews most of the legendary figures who have been the object of exposure and whose fate was significant. But here it is a question of children who were tested and not of abnormal children who were saved. "The idea that an infant should be sacrificed because, if it lived, it would bring misfortune is found, to the best of my knowledge, in only three legends: those of Oedipus, Paris, and Cypselus."[23] This feature is still not proof of the congenital deformity of Oedipus. But we already note that the mother of Cypselus was named Labda, that is, 'the lame,' and the condemnation of which the infant was the object resembles a sentence of exposure. All this is despite the embellishment of the story and the rescue that Herodotus describes in his text devoted to Cypselus. This parallel with Oedipus prompts Delcourt to write: "The legend of Oedipus, like that of Cypselus, is, I believe, transcribed from the habit of exposing deformed newborns at birth. . . . The unlucky deformity is then attributed to an ancestor, the grandfather, the mother, simple personifications of the illness which is at the very origin of the creation of the legend."[24] After summarizing the elements that are particular to

Oedipus, she continues: "I believe that in face of such a complex of facts and signifying names, it is difficult not to see in the Oedipus legend a mythic transcription of *apothesis.*" *Apothesis* was the term reserved for the exposure of infants born deformed, as distinct from *ekthesis,* which referred to fatal exclusion for other reasons as determined by the male head of the family.

This linguistic distinction invites a clarification. If it is true that the exposure of deformed infants cannot be separated from the overall practice of exposure, we should still not forget its specific nature. Here I would cite an article by Nicole Belmont.[25] Starting with the exposure of malformed and thus unlucky infants, she extends her view to include the very widespread rite of putting a newborn on the ground, a practice intended to give proof that the newly born belongs to humanity but which also introduces all the problems of socialization of the child, a problem that is different from that of its biological birth. Proceeding in this way, Belmont sees the clear distinction, which is also found in the practice of wet-nursing, between biological birth (and kinship) and social birth (and kinship). The rite of exposure to the earth is also a means to effect recognition by the father, and not only by the mother who gives birth. In short, the rite of deposition on the ground is polysemic, and, in the case where it extends to exposure/expulsion, it can be interpreted as a means for parents to avoid the threat that every infant poses for earlier generations, and thus prevent any hostile impulses toward the infant. All this seems to me as stimulating as it is oblivious of the radical nature of the exposure of deformed infants, which constitutes a radical form of exclusion. Moreover, the case of the abnormal must be associated with those who were excommunicated by virtue of their status as expiators, scapegoats. In both cases, we again find fear in the face of the anger of mysterious forces, anxiety over the unknown wrong, cause of the misfortune, and finally the desire to assign fault to a being who can be excluded. Where is the fault? Not immediately in the deformity, but it indicates that a lineage or a group is flawed. Oedipus, at his birth, seems to carry a counter-sign pointing to the particular and cursed destiny of his line. The different modalities of the exposure of Oedipus seem to confirm this interpretation.

The difficulty that attends a reading of ancient and legendary texts, and the contradictory elements of which they are composed, will permit only theses that edge into hypotheses. But studies such as the one that I have drawn on do, however, add considerable weight to an interpretation of the defect that Oedipus bears in terms of physical abnormality.

The harm-bringing infants that were exposed to the gods, but *not killed,* could be saved by these same gods to whom they were sacrificed. Such a rescue would be the equivalent of a consecration. Oedipus is in this category. Cursed and the bringer of misfortune, but untouchable and sacred.[26] This is the cultural message of the birth of Oedipus. The story begins there. Where does it end? With Sophocles and his *Oedipus at Colonus.* We could say that the end of the myth is death: the disappearance of Oedipus in a kind of divine aura. The aberrant infant, the sign of alterity, has become almost divine, as if marvelously carried off. Misfortune and marvel are united.

We come into the world poorly, but the exit is glorious. We are threatened, but there is salvation: Oedipus' lack is finally made good. From terrifying alterity (the deformity) to appeasing alterity (the disappearance of Oedipus), human life is not assured of its identity and stability, and society does not grant them. We are always other than what society made us and believes us to be. Society and social identity are relative. The disabled Oedipus undergoes trials that are intended to reveal the other side of society and of the individual. Tragically, Oedipus—Swollen-Foot—plays a role that will be assumed in a buffoon mode by the disabled in the entourage of medieval princes. Vulnerability, derision, nonreconciliation. Why? Because people cannot stand difference, otherness: one likes only one's like. Oedipus stands for difference rejected. He is doomed to incest (the love of the same) and to the violence that is its consequence: the execution of the father, the suicide of the wife-mother, the rifts and misfortunes among the children of incest. Difference *on earth* is not viable, is cursed, and it is rejected. But even while rejecting it, society is no less under the effects of antagonism, war, and blood. If society resolved the difference that malformation represents, it would make a decisive advance. Society would no longer live in the register of the same, between two exterior alterities, but would integrate the difference into its interior.

We can establish another correlation in the myth of Oedipus: between the two disabilities, that of birth (the pedal oedema) and that, inflicted, of blindness. Oedipus follows a trajectory between a malformation and a weakness, between a defect and a quasi-illness. Oedipus the king ends in this kind of blindness. From head to foot Oedipus is transpierced with disability. From one end of his life to the other, the law of difference and of lack weigh on him—to the precise extent that the law of the identical makes him suffer fatally. Like a sheet of paper, like a sign, Oedipus has two sides: intolerable difference and implacable mimesis.[27] Oedipus is the acme of anomaly; he is also the sharpest reflection of our normality. Our normality is our love of the same, and this normality is risk filled. The abnormality is Oedipus exposed at the beginning and exiled at the end. But over this course he discovers that desire for the same is destructive and that difference leads to a kind of paradise. Oedipus inverts society's functioning, just as he does that of kinship. He, the differing one, is victim of the identical, because the identical wishes to regulate the differing. The correlations between the two termini of the story are not everything. At the center of the account we find a kind of deformity, of abnormality: the Sphinx, who is presented as a monster. This winged woman-lion imposes a test, since a riddle must be solved. This test, which will qualify Oedipus to reign in Thebes, implicates his unlucky birth. Oedipus does not guess, he *knows*, as Delcourt rightly remarks, which oracle is about him! The riddle and his test implicate once again his difference, his aberration. The monstrousness of the Sphinx, who in certain texts of the Oedipus myth is his kinswoman (and who has been confused with Jocasta), also plays the same role: a bird of ill omen for the earth, a resistance that must be overcome, she also has an aspect that is almost divine. She, too, represents difference overcome, but signals the approaching drama of mimesis.

My analysis is consonant with that of René Girard,[28] with several important differences. As with Lévi-Strauss and in my own exposition, Girard places this question of the Other and the Same at the center of the tragic myth. In his eyes, Oedipus is the prototype for

difference negated. Difference represented by the father, who is not
and cannot be the son, whom Oedipus kills and replaces in the bed
of Jocasta, his mother. Like many critics, Girard attaches only an
allegorical value to the crooked walk. A kind of redundancy of the
oedipal destiny, which does not proceed according to established
rules, according to fundamental prohibitions (notably that against
incest). I shall return to this. Girard sees in Oedipus a figure of illusory and impossible difference. He did not respect the difference
between father and son, because difference is not the human lot.
The human lot is mimesis, the desire for the same, the desire for the
same desire as everyone else. In point of fact, Oedipus wishes to
reign over Thebes, like his father, and loves the same woman as his
father. The tragedy of Oedipus is "the production of the identical on
the basis of evanescent differences." The fact that there may be
seeking, even questing, for fruitful differences does not prevent us
from being *doomed* to this reproduction, this imitation, this assimilation. We are as if summoned to difference and to its acceptance, the
Other is a kind of horizon, but we cannot break the cycle of this
repetition of the identical, this fusion into the same. We cannot really
be son, brother, father, mother, without wanting to abolish these
differences. Up to this point Girard is fairly faithful to Freud and
shares in the pessimism over the setbacks that psychoanalysis has
suffered. But he supplements Freud. In fact, in his eyes the oedipal
tragedy is ultimately centered, not on incest, the slaying of the father, the misfortune of Oedipus, but on rivalry, fratricidal rivalry.
Everyone wants to be similar. And in point of fact, fratricidal killings
are very present in the myth. This is the indicator of the "mimetic
crisis" that interests Girard. We all want to have the same desires.
The outcome is violence, violence resolved by the expulsion of the
expiatory victim. And here, too, it is true that Oedipus is punished,
by his own hand, in becoming blind, and he leaves Thebes to become a wanderer. Oedipus plays the role of the scapegoat on whom
falls the social misfortune of the forced departure. Thebes emerges
from its crisis by ejecting this guilty party,[29] who is also just anyone at
all. Reconciliation does not occur, however, because Oedipus remains a victim who is ignorant of his status as such, a status that the

myth conceals. The function as expiatory victim remains the unthought part of the myth. This will no longer be the case in the New
Testament, where Jesus will understand, will denounce the violent
origins of society and in so doing will disassemble its mechanism.

The Freudian and Girardian interpretations, even though I am
not discussing them here in terms of the fruits they have borne, seem
to me to suffer from excessive disregard of these repeated disabilities.
Before carrying my argument through to its conclusion, I would emphasize that I do not at all claim to have exhausted the significance of
the oedipal myth. The tragic myth is and will remain the site of multiple readings. I am not in the least campaigning against the wonderful
literature on Oedipus, but am advancing a bit to the side, to display
yet another reading.

That the fate of this being, Oedipus, so vastly different from
others, should be imprisonment in the identical, so much is assured.
But that the story should "function entirely in terms of the identical" I
do not believe. Like Lévi-Strauss, for whom Girard's analysis served
only as an illustration of method, I shall leave this matter in the status
of a question asked, but I must admit to thinking that difference is
dealt with in real terms, and not simply through the mechanism of the
mimetic crisis and the sacrifice of the emissary victim.

As I said at the beginning, the Greek myth of Oedipus does not
end until *Oedipus at Colonus.* Oedipus does not end as a victim but as
a near-god. This has not been sufficiently noted. The wandering ceases
and the exclusion of the victim is to a venerable repose. The mechanism of emissary is particularly truncated and the exclusion itself is not
so victimizing as may seem. It is as much exclusion of the different that
too greatly wished to resemble, as it is ritual sacrifice. In fact, the
ritual aspect is hardly present. In the same way as the exposure of
deformed infants is hard to associate with ritual sacrifice, the expulsion
of Oedipus has only the appearance of a real sacrifice.

A more modest approach, it seems to me, but one just as significant, is to stay with the intolerable character of the difference, *starting
with the aberrant character of Oedipus.* It is the impingement of the
different on the identical that is not bearable. This different that tried
to ape the identical. It is possible to read the myth in a fashion inverse

to that of Girard: the incestuous quest, the imitation of the father (the Other) are thwarted by the one who represents alterity. Mimesis is denounced. The destiny of Oedipus is not so much to show that humanity is doomed to mimesis as it is to show its illusion. Oedipus figures the Other, even more than he does the Father. This figure is engaged by the myth in the mimetic quest in order to demonstrate its pathology just as much as to underline its inevitable character. Having fled, Oedipus returns to alterity, but as one glorified. Instead of saying with Girard that the tragic myth of Oedipus "introduces an illusory difference into the heart of the identical," I would say that it introduces an effective difference into the process of the identical. It is the identical that is illusory and that fails. As always, this kind of reversal of perspective is inaccurate to a certain degree, because identity and difference are always entangled in the Greek world. I wish to insist on the fact, however, that the Hellenic world is far from being under the sway of mimesis, and that difference obsesses it just as much. In the myth there is a denunciation of mimesis and of the agony to which it gives rise at the very heart of implacable fate. It is a light, not on the possibility of getting off without risk but on *the operation of difference.* Of course, difference is rejected and the influence of mimesis is impressively powerful. But the myth of Oedipus is also a protest against this imprisonment, a kind of cry for liberty. Oedipus remains different, having been so since birth, and his mimetic itinerary is the long account of the denial of this difference, by himself and by a society that is incapable of doing it justice. At the end of *Oedipus at Colonus* Oedipus pronounces terrible curses against his son Polynices, who reassumes the mimetic position in wishing at all cost to rule over Thebes in opposition to his brother, the usurper. Here we clearly seem to have returned to behavior directed by rivalry and a desire for the same. The curses of Oedipus can be interpreted as the designation of a victim: Polynices will be rejected. But, like the famous curses of Jesus against the victimizing violence of religion as represented by the Pharisees,[30] we can see a trace of clairvoyance concerning mimesis as a generator of violence. In this, Oedipus truly knows the ills that gnaw at humanity. Here he sets himself at the greatest distance from what was his own life.

We see the blind man leading others to the place of his disappearance, confiding to Theseus a secret not otherwise revealed. We know that the place and the name of his tomb are forbidden and hidden. And Theseus says, "As long as I observe this law, he [Oedipus] has assured me that misfortune will spare my country." Peace resides in the alterity of Oedipus, in his secret.

If we then agree to follow Sophocles to the end that he gives the myth of Oedipus in the Greek world, customary views of Oedipus may be modified. I insist on this finale because in my eyes, accustomed as they are to the structure of narrative texts, it is the correlative of the beginning of the myth. Oedipus is a being who signifies, in his disability, a very radical elsewhere and otherness. The trials and discursive agendas of Oedipus can be analyzed in many ways. I am making this analysis on my own, without forgetting the beginning and the end, that is, following the trajectory of a difference that is recognized only in the final act, but which is at work throughout the account.

Several remarks are necessary, before pursuing our inquiry through the literature of antiquity. I have tried to read the myth of Oedipus through the prism of the problem of the hero's deformity (and that of certain of his kin) and of the meeting with monstrosity.

I wanted to establish that we *may* read the myth by this path of access and that it would lend coherence.[31] I have omitted calling attention to many commentaries on this myth and many literary reworkings: in French, from Corneille to Robbe-Grillet, passing by Voltaire, Cocteau, Durand, and others. My interest here is not the myth of Oedipus as such but the problem of disability, addressed through it. I have tried to establish that for the Greeks physical deformity posed the very problem of their own human condition, a condition that seeks to seal the cracks of alterity, enveloped as it is in the desire for the same. But this is a condition that *recognizes* the question and casts a deeply suspicious eye on its desire for the identical, a tragic cry of protest. Greek culture was condemned to forget difference, but it was also aware of this. Thus, it knew that this difference would be its salvation. In point of fact, it sought to escape from this difference, but the wound was there, always raw.

One article in particular attests to the multiplicity of the readings of this myth, and adds to the store of questions raised by the literature on Oedipus.[32] Jean-Pierre Vernant takes as point of departure what Lévi-Strauss wrote in his most recent remarks on Oedipus: There is an intimate tie between lameness, which runs through the entire Greek mythic corpus, and the blocking of social communication on all levels (sexual, kin related, political). The author then attempts to juxtapose two texts: that of the legend of Oedipus and the historical one written by Herodotus about the tyrants of Corinth, the Cypselids, descended from Labda (*Labdabos*) the Lame. This is a successful juxtaposition. It does not interest me here as such, unless it is to add to the list of the malformed that we meet among the Greeks. Vernant comes to the conclusion that deformities, which lead to exposure or elimination, also give access to political power in the form of tyranny, that is, in the form of social disaggregation. The "lame" dynasties, like those of the Labdacids in Thebes or the Cypselids in Corinth, end in failure, because they "reject all the rules that in Greek eyes were at the foundation of communal life" (254). The tyrant removes himself from social interaction, like the original malformation that destabilizes power, sexuality, the succession of generations, and communication among kin. "The tyrant, both the equal of a god and a ferocious brute, incarnates in his ambivalence the mythic figure of the lame one, with his two opposing aspects: he goes beyond the human course because, rolling, moving swiftly and agilely, in all directions at once, he transgresses the limitations to which the one who 'walks straight' is subject. But his advance is also inferior to the normal mode of locomotion because, mutilated, off-balance, tottering, he proceeds by limping in his own particular way only to fall more completely at the end" (255). Given the vast learning we know Vernant to possess, this conclusion is inescapable by the end of his article and I shall not summarize it.

This study again underlines the importance, symbolic and real, of deformity and malformation. But, beyond that, the author recognizes that the problem is one of difference. A difference that fails, because it associates itself with a political form that operates outside the rules. The conclusions I have reached concerning Oedipus can be further shaded, because Oedipus, as I have said, ends well, even if it is in another world, and he hurls abuse at the fate of the Labdacids. It

remains true that the descendants of Oedipus are failures and this is
not insignificant when one recognizes the importance of lineage. But
the question of Oedipus is no less that of aberration and difference:
"How can a man participate in similitude . . . while three times becoming different in the course of his existence? How can the permanence of an order be sustained among creatures that are subject at
each age of their lives to a complete change of status? How can the
titles of king, father, husband, ancestor, son remain intact, unchange-
able when other people successively assume them and when one and
the same person is to be all of son, father, spouse, grandfather, young
prince, and old king in turn?" (243). This is the problem, the enigma of
Oedipus, well posed. It calls into question stability, permanence, the
identical, and identity. Disability defies order, and order is prey to
disorder, which has a primordial and radical character.[33]

To conclude this discussion of the oedipal myth I shall quote
Vernant. In answer to the question of what the tragic in Sophocles'
play consists, he replies that the duality of Oedipus' being is at the
heart of the tragic. I hope that I may be allowed a rather lengthy
quotation, which goes to the heart of our subject. Why say less well
what another has already expressed perfectly?

> Even the very name of Oedipus contributes to these effects of
> reversal. Ambiguous as it is, it carries within itself the same
> enigmatic character that marks the entire tragedy. Oedipus is
> the man with the swollen foot (*oîdos*), a disability that recalls the
> cursed child, rejected by its parents, exposed to die in the wilder-
> ness. But Oedipus is also the man who knows (*oîda*) the riddle of
> the foot, who succeeds in solving, without getting it backwards,
> the 'oracle' of the sinister prophetess, the Sphinx of the dark
> song. And this knowledge makes ironic the presence of the for-
> eign hero in Thebes, establishes him on the throne in place of the
> legitimate kings. The double meaning of *Oidipous* is found at the
> center of the name itself in the contrast between the two first
> syllables and the third. *Oida*, I know, one of the principal words
> in the mouth of the triumphant Oedipus, of Oedipus the tyrant.
> *Pous*, the foot, the mark imposed from birth on him whose fate is
> to end as he began, in exclusion, resembling the wild animal that

his footstep causes to flee, the one whose foot isolates him from
humans in the vain hope of escaping from the oracles, pursued by
the curse of the terrifying foot because he infringed the laws
sacred to the elevated foot, and henceforth incapable of getting
his foot out of the misfortunes into which he precipitated himself
by raising himself to the summit of power. The whole tragedy of
Oedipus is as if contained in the wordplay to which the riddle of
his name lends itself.

And a bit later in the same text: "The exposed infant may be a discard
that society wants to be rid of, a deformed monster or a base slave. But
he may also be a hero with an exceptional destiny. Saved from death,
triumphant in the test that is imposed on him from birth, the exile is
revealed as the elect, invested with supernatural power" (38).

Hephaestus . . . and Others
Oedipus is not the only famous deformed person in classical literature.
Disability reaches the gods themselves in the person of Hephaestus.[34]
As with Oedipus, we do not know exactly what his disability was, nor
how it occurred. Crippled in both legs from birth? Twisted foot? Dwarf
and bow-legged? There is no certainty. Born of a woman without the
intervention of a father? Son of Zeus and Hera? Fathered by a giant
who raped his mother Hera? We are not sure. But that he is disabled
and that his birth was special, there is no doubt. He suffered the fate of
unlucky infants: he was expelled and thrown from Olympus by Zeus,
but in this case not at birth. His expulsion is always connected with his
disability. In addition, Delcourt very judiciously distinguishes between his disability, which is from birth, and his deformity, which is
the result of the fall. "The disability and deformity of Hephaestus have
differing origins. The former is the price paid by the magician to
acquire his art; the latter is both the symbol of the most awesome
powers and the most efficacious means to hold them at bay should they
become aggressive." In this magical world, everything is done back-
wards (feet the wrong way around!) and this "corresponds to the belief
that sees in the monstrous and terrifying object a power capable both
of calling up the most dangerous forces and of checking them" (131). It

is from his birth and his accident that Hephaestus draws his magic power. He is primarily a magician, manipulating the arts and talismans in the fashion of a shaman. Many magician-gods, beyond Greece, are mutilated: Varuna is crippled, Tyr has lost a hand, Odin is one-eyed.

Rejected because of his anomaly, Hephaestus then harnesses extraordinary abilities. We find here the same two faces of deformity: ostensibly eliminated, it may return equipped with supernatural forces. This dimension of magician, which is undeniable, does not, however, determine the identity of Hephaestus. In the *Iliad* he is found as cup-bearer, then as master of metals and magical objects, finally as the Lord of Fire. It would seem that one could synthesize his activities and role in the mastery of the *bond*. He intervenes to enchain or to unfetter. The god of tying and untying, he has also become the artisan god, the patron of those who transform. In short, along with his deformity, and doubtless because of it, Hephaestus can lay claim to the occult, artistic power of the craftsman. He is not associated with power as understood in the sociopolitical sense, but he is *powerful*. His inherent weakness opens for him the domain of mysterious efficacy. The disability excludes him from a public role, from the structure of power (let us not forget the failure of Oedipus). But disability is in collusion with the whole underside of appearances and of the established; it allows his participation in another, secret face of things. Disability is not admitted to everyday organization; it is not *integrated* in that sense. But it opens the door to the arcane. The deformed being could play only an exceptional and not a current role, but he does play a role. The disabled god is left to his alterity; usually it is destabilizing and terrifying, but he has been given a function that is indicative, disruptive, subversive, prestigious, theurgical. His fate is not in the least trivialized and, as an individual, he suffers most atrociously at times, but his alterity tears a certain veil that masks our ordinary arrangements. In the final analysis, the disabled person is never considered an *individual* who ought to be able to live among others; he is always considered a sign, a collective one, "good to think about," as Lévi-Strauss would say, "good to worry about," I would add.

Hephaestus has been made a kinsman of Philoctetes, another aberrant figure. Solidarity in marginality. Philoctetes is not disabled from birth. As owner of the bow and arrows of Hercules, he makes his way to Troy. Stopped at Chryse, he is bitten on the foot by a serpent. His wound gives off an intolerable odor of rotting. The heads of the army that he is accompanying abandon him alone on the island of Lemnos where he lives in terrible, solitary exile. Since Ulysses lacks Philoctetes' skill and the power of his arrows, he tries to get his weapons by a trick while leaving Philoctetes to his misery. In the end the good conscience of Ulysses' envoy causes the trap to fail and, on the recommendation of Hercules himself, Philoctetes embarks to join the battle, assured of a cure and of victory. Such is the content of the play by Sophocles.

Here it is a question of abandoning the sick person, the wounded warrior, the accidentally disabled man. It is a drama of solitude and rejection because the hero has been rendered powerless. But akin to Hephaestus, Philoctetes possesses a kind of secret weapon from Hercules.

Disability and other powers are again linked. Philotectes, rejected by the organization and the sociopolitical enterprise personified in Ulysses, finds himself endowed with a strength and efficacy that come from a god. The same relationship between nonintegration and superior role is again seen. Philotectes is a new representative of the Other, excluded but advanced, rejected but exalted. Myth always works on two levels: the political and social level, where there is no room for aberration, and the magical and collective level, where there exists an eminent function for aberration in the service of the human community.

As for the aberrancy of Hermaphrodite, although it poses a whole series of questions that will not be treated here, it seems to offer new but consonant proof of what I have just said. The figure with double sex, with a body both masculine and feminine, is fairly common in the pantheons of various cultures. For the Greco-Roman world it should first be stated that sexual ambivalence was considered an anomaly, the most dangerous of all and the most monstrous. "When an infant was born with the real or apparent signs of hermaphroditism, the entire community judged itself threatened by the anger of the gods."[35] These newborns were exposed, like those I have already written about. Many children were exposed (or drowned or burned) because their sex was uncertain. And yet we find that Hermaphrodite (Hermes plus Aphrodite) was the object of a very widespread cult. Even if the origin of the cult of Hermaphrodite is correlated with a reduction in the practice of exposure, the central question remains when we consider Greek culture as a whole. Moreover, the elimination of infants of doubtful sex persisted until the end of antiquity: Plutarch testifies to this. How does it happen that we find at the same time a rejection of bisexuality in perceived maleficent deformations and the cult of a bisexual divinity? No doubt for the same reason that we find a god, Hephaestus, both misshapen and magician. Hermaphrodite protects sexual unions and births. He/she is the figure of the impossible: androgyny. And androgyny is itself the figure of what is no longer different, of what fuses. There is no longer man and woman; man and woman are the same, are identical.[36] Hermaphrodite wields a power over sexuality because she/he is not sexually normal. While on the concrete level of the everyday, the biological, the social, sexual anomaly is expelled and sent back to the gods, on the religious and mythic level (which is also the collective level), the difference is sacralized and becomes the site of a power that has influence over love affairs. But this difference, as I have just said, figures the identical. We find again the same obvious riddle as with Oedipus. Hermaphrodite signifies to us that love is implacably doomed to the search for the same, for mimesis, for fusion.

As concerns the Greek world, I must reiterate my rather abrupt statement. For Plato, particularly in his dialogue *The Symposium*, love can also recognize differences and is played out in a plural fashion, man and man, man and woman, woman and woman. The desire for a unity that goes beyond oppositions and differences, however, along with the myth of the androgyne, dominates discourse. Moreover, Hermaphrodite, at the same time as he/she illustrates the tendency of love to merge, denounces this fusion and mimesis by *protecting* love affairs from a similar move to common identity, just as he/she watches over unlucky bisexual births.[37] Like Oedipus, she/he shows to just what degree our desire for the same—and our aversion to the different (sexual in this instance)[38]—extends, but she/he casts an uneasy, critical glance on it; he/she checks it. Moreover, as Delcourt points out, there is a latent androgynism in Greek art, a constant ambivalence about bodies: Hermaphrodite carries this to the limit. This reveals the typical character that Hermaphrodite assumes in the classical mentality. The highest values are attributed to Hermaphrodite, but he/she stigmatizes characteristics that are not tolerable in empirical everyday life. Delcourt is aware of this when she writes that "an idea may be translated by symbols, provided that these symbols do not become so precise as to coincide with concrete reality" (77). Social order no more permits hermaphroditism than it tolerates lameness or a webbed hand. Social order recognizes the challenge of alterity yet cannot accept it.

To accept my analysis one would have to distance oneself somewhat from the development that Greek and Roman thought would undergo, particularly among the philosophers. This is quite evident in the case of the myth of the androgyne. In fact, the symbol of the androgyne is almost always speculatively interpreted only in the register of the dream of *unity,* a preexistent unity that the world has left behind or a unity to be remade, beyond separation. In this kind of reflection there is hardly any room for the fertile paradox that I am trying to identify. Hermaphrodite is a projection of what is most desirable, even what is most complete. But if we are directed in our thinking by the contrast between social practice and the oppositional religious figure of Hermaphrodite (as well as by that of Oedipus or Hephaestus), then we would have to take this contrast into account. It seems to me that the path that opens is the one I have marked out: difference is intolerable in the here and now, but it remains the object of a nostalgia that destabilizes the received and inevitable order, which in turn experiences its derision and arbitrariness. Just as the Greek world is characterized not only by reason and clarity, but also by irrationality and the duping of reason, so on the level that interests me it is not characterized by a unilateral search for identity and mimesis, but by the other and by separation as well.

To conclude with a schematic presentation similar to those that I have proposed at the end of other chapters, I summarize what seem to me the major organizing oppositions in classical thought on the problem of disability.

Sociobiological level (or isotopy)

differing/identical
└─────────────┘

CONFORMITY

– –

EXCLUSION (cannot be situated)

┌─────────────┐
threatening/exalting

Religious level (or isotopy)

We see the contrast with the biblical system: for the latter it is
primarily a question of biological integrity, which the ethical-religious
point of view can situate but not necessarily integrate or treat. Here it
seems to me that the emphasis is as much on the social problem as on
the biological one. It is conformity that is the interrogator. The religious level (and not the ethical) does not situate nonconformity: able
only to fear it or give it extraordinary status, it is obliged to exclude it,
in the most radical way possible.

4

The System(s) of Charity

When we finish reading the historians of the Middle Ages, our disappointment is great. This is not the fault of the historians. Is it simply because we stand before one of the silences of history? Can this silence to be broken by future works? Most certainly. But there is perhaps a more indicative kind of silence, one that asks the question: why is there not more historical discourse still to be realized?

I shall get to this in some detail, to lend support to the saying, so pertinent here: "We only talk about those not present." In other words, if the historical account is so brief, it is perhaps because the disabled, the impaired, the chronically ill were spontaneously part of the world and of a society that was accepted as being multifaceted, diversified, disparate. The kind of social eugenics that was to be the fate of recent society had not yet emerged. Normality was a hodgepodge, and no one was concerned with segregation, for it was only natural that there should be malformations. This was more than tolerance; it was real life, with which one compromised as best one could, without wishing to change it by various techniques and various treatments, and without wishing to exclude it either. There was an acceptance, at times awkward, at times brutal, at times compassionate, a kind of indifferent, fatalistic integration, without ideology but also without confrontation. This would have been the general attitude of medieval society toward disability.[1] It is true that the silence of which I spoke, which goes beyond the present limitations of historical works, makes us pause and reflect.

In addition, we know that the Middle Ages were very traditional in all sorts of areas; they borrowed a great deal and repeated even more. In speaking on the subject of monsters and deformities, Claude Kappler writes: "The intellectual attitude is little inclined to renew itself in this respect. Until the fifteenth century there are few creations or original thoughts on the subject. . . . We have to wait for the sixteenth century. . . . Ambroise Paré will apply himself to the matter."[2]

As a consequence, this inquiry would come to a quick close if it were true that, for the Middle Ages as a whole, physical aberrancy like all monstrosities was a "normal anomaly" in the face of which there was neither revulsion, nor terror, nor treatment: it was a simple occasion to do good and to praise God for the infinite diversity of his creation and the mysterious harmony of his design (Saint Augustine).

It would be frivolous, however, to renounce our inquiry so summarily. There is an abundant, even overflowing, secondary literature from the last few years concerning the poor and poverty in the medieval period. A new question then arises: did the disabled and impaired of various kinds simply melt into the crowd of the poor? If so, then their history would have been written.[3] And if this is not the case, we are again referred back to a meditation on silence.

What can this history of the poor tell us? I shall not give a scholarly summary; anyone can get and read a book on the subject. What is so remarkable is that these studies are in agreement in breaking the medieval period up into stages, where society passed from dark and brutal years tempered by charity to a time of spiritual and social dignity and valorization, until the revolt of the poor and their invasion of the larger community. After this, in the neoclassical age in France there began what might be called, after Foucault, "the great confinement." This massive consensus, even if it is open to discussion, is remarkable in the following respect: there were several subsystems in the social treatment of the poor during the Middle Ages.

Some will think this a flat observation, given the vast temporal span that is considered. Its banality, however, invites us to interpret certain silences in different ways than before. Yet even among written sources, there is still more about disability to be considered. We begin with a little anthology of remarks.

If we move to the close of the Middle Ages, we meet phrases such as the following: "these beggars, prostitutes, thieves, cutpurses, by vocation or by chance (students and wandering clerics), these disabled and sick, real or simulated, these blind men and prostituted women constituted, in certain town quarters, virtual worlds unto themselves, cohesive communities with their own laws and language, their own leaders."[4]

Here then are the impaired in the very middle of the Cours des Miracles (the city area frequented by these groups), misery and the underworld at the same time. It is easy to understand why they also figure in the list of frightening realities: "The potential guilty parties, against whom collective aggression may be diverted, are primarily strangers, travelers, the marginalized, and all those who are not fully integrated into the community, either because they are not willing to accept its beliefs—the case of the Jews—or because it was necessary for obvious reasons to reject them to the periphery of the group—the case of lepers—or, finally, simply because they came from somewhere else. . . . In fact, lepers were accused in 1348–50 of having spread the Black Death."[5] The phenomenon of fear, fundamental to the end of the Middle Ages and the Renaissance, encompassed the disabled and ended in their sequestration in the almshouse (*l'hôpital général*), as well in the first appearance of the concept of putting all these people to work.[6]

Undistinguished at the end of the medieval period from all the marginalized and indigent, both horrifying and dangerous, who would revolt and then be put aside and regulated in the cities—even if some rare theologians speak of the rights of the poor[7]—the disabled were no less undistinguished at the dawn of the Middle Ages from the economically weak. "The category of disabled and sick seems numerous and everywhere present. Gregory of Tours, Fortunatus, and the lives of saints mention many feebleminded, leprous, and blind people, the last-named in large groups."[8] From remarks such as this, historians have inquired into the health conditions of society to see whether these disabilities are due to malnutrition and deficient hygiene, initially and especially as they affected the impoverished and squalid levels of society. If we make a probe into the central Middles Ages, at the apogee of this vast civilization, the view of the poor changes, but the disabled remain mixed in among them. In fact, Francis of Assisi introduces a novelty: "Esteem for the poor and the afflicted by reason of their spiritual value and their essential humanity, and no longer simply as the still servile instruments of the salvation of the rich."[9] Nonetheless this same Francis of Assisi, the first sign of whose conversion was to kiss a *leper* (who transformed himself into the figure of Christ), saw in him the representative of all the poor whom he loved so much. We do not find in his biography a rigorous distinction between the poor and the disabled, even though Saint Francis does constitute a turning point in medieval thought.

Whether we look to the beginning of the Middle Ages or to the end or to the central centuries, everywhere "the sick and the disabled are caught in the infernal machinery of pauperization."[10] We meet them on the pilgrimage routes: "As for the blind, the deaf, the mildly paralyzed who could move, they obstinately sought cures by travelling to new sites whose sudden fame drew great crowds."[11] In his paintings Brueghel places amputees and the simple among the mass of the poor who were beggars in public places.[12] And yet, despite this striking mixture of the poor and the disabled, we can note, by way of a historian's remark, another perspective. With regard to the hospices created in the fourteenth and fifteenth centuries, we read: "All kinds of the sick are taken in there, *with the exception of* lepers, the lame, one-armed, and blind, who by virtue of their incurable disabilities cannot be considered truly sick. On the other hand, pregnant women without means were given shelter,[13] because 'three categories of persons are admitted into the hospices: the poor, pilgrims, and especially the sick.' "[14] The disabled were not always assimilated to the poor and the sick. Moreover, throughout the Middle Ages there was treatment for lepers, a treatment that was not comparable to that for the poor.

Lepers often constituted a kind of urban community of their own, but it was not characterized by poverty. Excluded as a prophylactic measure (and this in itself is a question to be readdressed), they became a kind of new order. Entry into a leper house was comparable to the entry into the religious life[15] and the organization of these ghettos was modeled on that of a monastery, even down to the architecture. The leprosaria were beneficiaries of legacies, there was a chapel, a priest, etc. Without doubt, all the disabled could not be accorded the

tance: the established powers are challenged in order to be over-thrown and replaced. The guiding concepts are destruction and re-placement but without that detachment that was the special feature of the Middle Ages and which was less subversive but perhaps more lucid.

Moreover, the medieval monster—those races of monsters that were called real, that appeared on the maps of the Middle Ages—is not simply an ethical reminder and a means to exorcize fear. Like the fool or the disabled person in the company of the mighty of this world, the medieval monster first teaches us that the world is composed of the same and of the different, that it is essentially variegated. Saint Augustine discusses monstrosity in *The City of God.* In addition to a number of justifications for these bizarre beings, he sets the tone for the entire Middle Ages: God created prolifically and esthetically. In order to create a fine cloth, threads of different colors must be mixed, contrasts must be established. The cause and the role of monsters is the glorification of God. "The song of the universe cannot give up its entire secret: harmonies and discordances, dissonances and conso-nances battle with one another in full agreement according to the principle of great medieval polyphony."[22]

Recent writing on the monsters of the Middle Ages reveals many other aspects as well.[23] The conclusion of a book like Kappler's is a profusion of significations, aspects, and divisions. But for our subject, this kind of study can be dangerous: the monsters and the disabled are so closely associated that a reader might imagine referring the question of physical aberration to that of monstrosity. Certainly, the monstrous can include human deformity. In his typology of monsters and marvels Kappler—and this is no criticism—combines human and animal mon-sters or, even more frequently, monsters both human and bestial. His classification encompasses not only what is real deformity but also imagi-nary configurations. Monstrosity in the Middle Ages, for many think-ers, was akin to artistic or imaginative creation. Indeed, Kappler de-votes a very interesting section to the relationship between monsters and language in order to show how monstrosity was often an effect of narrative or of the literary image. In travel literature, in cartography, authors proceeded blithely to amplify their received accounts, even to invent passages out of whole cloth. Monsters must in part be referred to fable. The medieval world is stuffed, saturated with amazing things. I recognize the thrilling aspect of research into the signification, functioning, and social role of this incredible population. In the following, I shall not fail to cite them since studies of monsters give us information very pertinent to the question of disability. This is not surprising, since the *notion* of monster is necessarily related to that of disability. But I would emphatically underscore the deceptive character of any attempted merger of the two phenomena.

The impression that before the end of the French classical age— the seventeenth and early eighteenth centuries—there was no specific vision of the disabled, no more than any special treatment, is not so justified as might be thought. If, to a great extent, the disabled are included among the poor, they are distinguished from them in certain respects. If they are associated with marginality, they are unknown to the mythology of a localized Elsewhere; if they are at times grouped with dangerous people, they are not reduced simply to this status, even during the troubled period that followed the Black Death and during the mass wandering at the end of the medieval period. In relation to these three groups we begin to wonder whether there is not a precise place to be considered, in the hollow, the crack, in-between. Beyond these figures, so important for the Middle Ages—the beggar, the monster, the criminal—lies the silhouette of the disabled, borrowing features from the other three all at the same time or successively, and yet sharply contoured, taking us down into the depths of as yet unthought social ideas.

Because there are texts! As I have already stated emphatically, social constructions are as important as effective practices in representing a society. Even more: these representations of a phenomenon are just as much part of reality as "what happens." Even if what happens is not discourse, how we talk about things, discourse is just as important for social reality. Moreover, discourse often differs from the praxis of the moment, but at one time or another informs it even more than earlier praxis. There is a false opposition between discourse and the real. The realism of common sense is not so real as one thinks. Discourse is nowhere else than in the real. Is praxis itself anything but part of the discursive?

To discourse then. Especially since the historians' history is mute. Once and for all it is time to show that discourse tells us more than do the facts. What are the facts of discourse?

From Zotikos to Francis of Assisi

Poorhouse Charity and the Ethics of Almsgiving

Zotikos was martyred at the dawn of the Christian era for having cared for lepers. Francis of Assisi began his life as a convert by kissing lepers, at the end of a medieval age under the sign of almsgiving, at the beginning of an age that glorified the poor.

Zotikos is offered here as the paradigm for early Christianity not only because he lived in Byzantium (later Constantinople) during the reign of Constantine but also because the text with the legend of his life is of primary significance. All historians of Constantinople, like all historians of poverty, call attention to Zotikos. He was not the only one to succor the sick and disabled. Public establishments such as alms-houses or hospices, almost like communities of the poor, did exist and were close in organization to the monasteries, although lay, popular, and unstable. These institutional forms did not last.[24] A thinker like John Chrysostom would disapprove of them.[25] They were a source of disorder and risked escaping from the control of the church. The organization of charity for the poor and disabled would move in the direction of a kind of assumed care for social outcasts. "The church, rich in its own right (since Constantine), more or less controlled the world of the rich and took charge of the world of the poor: it structured this economic situation and social problem into a system."[26] This would be the system of foundations where, through the intermediary of the church, the generosity of the rich was transformed into the subsistence of the poor. We can even see, in the way in which the church would come to aid the poor, the passage from an economic system based on gifts to a system of exchange.[27] We should add that the ongoing discourse of the Middle Ages claimed that the rich assured their salvation by giving alms to the poor and it thus posited the necessity of the poor for such salvation. The world is inevitably constituted of rich and poor, and the salvation of some proceeds by way of charity toward others. The struggle to eradicate poverty is not a social priority in the medieval period. The universe of thought is an ethical universe and not a political one, and hardly technological at all. We can then understand that poverty might find itself borne to the highest rank among human and spiritual values.

In Zotikos we can see the rupture between the society of charity that would develop and the religious world of Greek or Jewish antiquity. Whether the person who is celebrated is the historical one or not, and whether the account of his life[28] is completely legendary or not are of no importance in this context. The text of his biography points up the opposition between two systems. I have spoken of the exposure of deformed infants and of the social constructions that justified it. Here, Zotikos, who founds a leprosarium with money diverted from Constantine, goes directly against the wishes of the emperor, according to the text: "All those whose body is ruined by leprosy and who struggle against that disease which is called sacred he ordains to be driven from the city or even to be thrown into the depths of the sea" (75).[29] In so doing, Constantine shows that he belongs to the world of antiquity and its practice of exposure, the fatal exclusion. Zotikos does the opposite. On Mount Olivet, where they would have perished in the presence of the gods, in atonement before divine anger, Zotikos "granted them all his attention, readying huts made of cut branches . . . preparing potions for them." The symbol of the passage from one mental world to another was the leprosy of the daughter of Constans, Constantine's successor, who was condemned to death by drowning and whom Zotikos conducted to his leper house, saving her from this form of exposure. Once Zotikos had been martyred, Constans repented of his actions and constructed a hospice, endowing it with both personal and imperial resources. Zotikos shook the classical world. And here is the text, flat on a first reading and the very antithesis of the earlier system: "The primary and urgent mission of doing good to the sick who are there, of coming to their aid and of responding generously to their needs; knowing that God cares for them as for none other, God to whom they seek to offer mercy by their intervention, for they have need of mercy before the day of judgment" (83). The discourse of the life of Zotikos is a pivotal account.

Let us further consider this text. Children were abandoned in antiquity. This text speaks of providing for them. Care becomes a primary and urgent mission. Before, it was primary, in the sense of a first necessity, and urgent, in the sense of not tolerating delay, to expose the misshapen. Admittedly, the text of this biography deals with the sick and not with the deformed. But in the house founded by Zotikos were people of all kinds, in particular lepers. Because God was concerned for them, the text continues, while earlier gods protected society at their expense. In the world of antiquity they had to be removed, returned to the gods who might let them perish—the usual case in concrete terms—or grant them an exceptional destiny, in the world of myth. Here God is solicitous of them, and society is obliged to take care of them. Difference is always at the heart of the problem and of its solution, but it is given a wholly new treatment: divine and human mercy. It is no longer a question of culpability, as announced by the deformed person, weighing on the group. It is no longer a matter of returning to the gods the being who symbolized their anger. Mercy must be rendered to God with a view to an ethical judgment, while, earlier, atonement had to be offered to the gods in order to ward off the punishment of misfortune. To me, it is striking that this text, to whose select and particular vocabulary M. M. Aubineau calls attention, should be the exact antithesis of Greco-Roman practice, as still represented by Constantine himself. The symmetry is too great to be the result of chance. The more so, since the text appears at the beginning of organized Christianity, in the capital of the new empire whose ruler was a convert. Zotikos stands in opposition to the emperor, who represented the succession of the world of antiquity, despite his conversion. The entire situation and context has a bridging value: why has this text been chosen? Zotikos inaugurates the system of charity.

Zotikos, the Christian martyr, is the heir to the Gospels. He bears witness to a new attitude toward misfortune and suffering, that of

Christ, of which I have written earlier. Rejecting the system of Jewish religious prohibitions, like that of the pagans with its divinatory content, he heralds a way of life in which both ideas and behavior will be shaken and topple. The difference represented by the poor and disabled is no longer the counterweight of an invading mimesis: it becomes part of the everyday with which we must live and which we must see as coming to us from God in order to sanctify us. It is no longer a question of giving back to the divinity but of accepting a gift.

Was this tolerable? Did society not risk being shaken to its religious foundations? The patristic period attempted to give a response to these questions. Saint Augustine, as I have already said, tried to reduce substantially the abnormal and terrifying character of anomaly. In his theological and aesthetic perspective, he effects a double operation: he exonerates God of these malformations and he relieves humanity of its fear. Dissimilarity is for him neither a chance event nor a punishment but the sign of the inscrutable grandeur of the Creator. Position yourselves, he proposes, for a view of the whole. In the vast plan or design of God there exists a diversity, an infinite variety to make the world into a harmony that is beyond our control. On the level of detail you may find that something is an error of God, a failure, but this simply means that you are missing the great architectonics, the global vision. Moreover, more prosaically, Saint Augustine believed in the existence of races of monsters, somewhere at the geographical limit of the human world: the human monster represented an exception justified by this existence, which contributed to the symphony of creation.[30] As seen by our limited intelligence, deformities are connected to faults in the created order but seen through an effort of deeper intelligence they form part of a global *beauty.*

Augustine would not be supported in all quarters and monstrosity would be associated with Satan and his demons. Yet this did not prevent Augustine from decisively integrating anomaly into the normal, and difference into the *order* of things. It is no longer a scandal, that is, a hindrance that rocks the understanding of the sublunar world. This idea of the scandalous can also serve as a red thread for many reflections on difference.[31] In the New Testament Jesus invites his disciples to move beyond the scandalous, to overcome what stands as obstacle to the contemplation of the Father. Saint Augustine is faithful to this Gospel lesson.

What then will the disabled person be? Someone to stimulate charity since he is part of creation and is no longer intrinsically associated with sin, fault, culpability, or with the anger of the gods, or with nonintegrable difference. This will be the constantly reiterated message of the church fathers, often the founders of charitable works and hospices. But this is not to say that the disabled, congenital or adventitious, are integrated in the contemporary sense of the term; rather, they no longer symbolize metaphysical and biological difference that questions the species and the social unit. They now constitute a difference to be loved, helped, aided, furthered. They will continue to be indicators of another world, not in the emotional register of religious fear but in that of spirituality and morality. These two are very distant one from the other; in the former case, we meet a behavioral praxis of radical rejection, in the latter, conduct based on fundamental acceptance. In the strictly religious universe, deformity frightens objectively by the danger that it represents; in an ethical and charitable universe, it may still cause subjective fear, but it becomes the touchstone for submission to a greater order.

On the practical level this new view would for centuries result in nothing more than alms, either individually given or in the form of institutionalized works of charity. These two alternatives should not be understood exactly in the modern sense; almsgiving was a very noble activity and, in the economic system of these centuries when feudalism was being established, it was a means of redistributing wealth. Alms was not only the coin that one slid into the beggar's hand; often it rose to very substantial amounts, in the form of rents paid regularly or in a lump sum, in the form of foundations and legacies. All charitable action was thus financed by the rich, who could be nobles of the courts or kings and emperors themselves (at times drawing on public funds, at times private). In short, almsgiving was part of the system. As for institutionalized activity on behalf of the needy, it too should not be imagined in modern fashion: it provided accommodation and little else. The hospices, which became very numerous after Constantine and were characteristic of the Christian era,[32] made up a network of very small establishments attached to and run by a monastery, a bishopric, or a lord. Thus a single term (Fr. *hôpital*) covers an extremely varied reality throughout the period.

But it should be recognized that the primary problem of the long period of the high Middle Ages was not deformity. The illnesses of infancy, accidents during pregnancy or delivery made for their own natural selection. Society was not obliged to deal with elevated numbers of disabled, as today. Sickness concerned the period in a different way, principally in the phenomenon of epidemics. Without population mobility in the early period, epidemics were limited in geographical scope but nonetheless devastating. Once trade and travel were extended, epidemics would become terrifying, decimating, ending in the notorious plagues of the fourteenth and fifteenth centuries: bubonic plague, cholera, rabies. We shall return to this at a later point. Histories of illness and medicine, when they deal with this period, do not inform us on the question of disability.

The only thing we can state with confidence is that people of all kinds were to be found in the *Maison Dieu* (the hospices were called "Houses of God"), always with the exception of lepers and, at times, the incurable and paralyzed.[33] The "mad" were often imprisoned and it would not be until 1375 in Hamburg that the first specialized asylum was created.[34] Then in Spain, Italy, and France this example would be followed, although in these more Latin countries the developmentally retarded and their assets were long placed in the custody of a guardian. The insane poor would be in the care of the family, the lord, or the police. The blind, who often had rather more prestige, be it only by reason of the Gospels, would benefit from a number of asylums even before the celebrated foundation of Les Quinze-Vingts by Saint Louis, which was actually more of a refuge than a hospice. Nor should we forget all the aid that was provided to homes. Much help and assistance remained on a personal and individualized basis. The mother of Saint Bernard, the pious Alicia, recrossed the countryside in search of the *disabled* and indigent. Many saints did the same thing. For the disabled, Saint Rosa of Viterbo should particularly be named.

On the other hand, the difficulty of knowing just where the disabled were continues for the entire medieval period. Even in the fourteenth century we still see Jeanne of Valois stating that one should practice the "seven works of mercy" in the hospices. One of these seven works was to visit the *infirmes*, although at the time the French word meant only the weak and not the crippled. The rules of the almshouses, however, at times excluded paralytics (as was often to prove the case) or bedridden persons incapable of working; more frequently, the lame, one-armed, and blind were excluded, since their incurable disability did not constitute a sickness in the narrow sense of the word.[35] But there was a great deal of indecision in the matter.

For the early Middle Ages as for the period that will begin toward the end of the twelfth century, the categorization of various impairments and disabilities is far from clear, no clearer than the social treatments adopted on their behalf. Not only is disability not the primary problem, as I have noted, but it is neither inventoried, nor excluded, nor organized, nor viewed in any special way: it is simply there, part of the great human lot of misery. It too deserves mercy.

Mystical Ethics: When the Disabled Becomes Christ

No historian would this deny this statement by a colleague: "The Franciscan movement was a great religious phenomenon that, more than any of the other mendicant orders, shook, marked, informed the whole of Christian society in the thirteenth century."[36] My agreement stops perhaps at this generality, so complex is the Franciscan question. Who was the saint from Assisi? An innovator, even a bold challenger, or a submissive orchestrator? What did he want? A simple fraternity, more lay than clerical, subverting the idea of power and property, or an Order, new but without an objective much more precise than personal conversion? What was the historical impact? A real upheaval in spiritual, theological, and social thought, or a fine flight of fancy, the effects of which were damped scarcely fifty years after the death of Poverello, the "Poor Little One"?

Obviously, I shall not enter into the labyrinth of debates that are periodically raised by the spiritual family that succeeded Francis and by historians. The secondary literature on the Franciscan question is among the most ample there is. Why choose the Franciscan event as indicative of a turning point that concerns my topic? Because the relationship with poverty, under the aspect of the concreteness of poverty, underwent undeniable change in the circles around Francis of Assisi. From poverty I have an entry into a new mentality concerning aberrancy and marginality. But, as is always the case in history, it is not a single person or event that counts. What counts is the historical cleavage that stimulated a great and intense germination. This caesura must be given reference points and a quite visible expression, and Francis of Assisi does this. He joins the lineage of a multitude of poverty movements, marked with the names of Robert d'Arbrissel, Peter Valdo, Armand of Brescia, Durandus, and so on.[37] Similarly, Francis reflects, on his spiritual level, new social divisions. It was not without purpose that I cited Le Goff earlier. This historian shows, through the study of the Franciscan vocabulary, that the dominant distinction for the pauper from Assisi is not the usual division of orders (those who pray, those who fight, those who labor) or the ecclesiastical division between clerics and laymen. Mixing together several paradigms, he would see society as a set of nonhierarchical categories, preferentially resting on two parties: the well-off, powerful, and educated, and the poor, disenfranchised, and ignorant. Without in the least making Francis of Assisi a precursor of Karl Marx, we can legitimately see in him one who, from the partisan struggles of the Italian cities of his time, perceived one great divide and had the dream of eliminating the opposition between superior and inferior. Le Goff can only note the social failure of this undertaking that was not, however, consciously a militant movement, but spiritual preaching. In fact, the perspective tended toward pauperism, the inverse of the capitalist society that would follow. An "economy of poverty," in the words of Joseph Folliet, was comprised in the vision of Francis of Assisi at a time when a merchant economy and then economies of surplus and consumption were in the process of development.

But on the level of the attitude toward the poor, Francis left his mark. The poor became more than persons to be aided, they became charged with the greatest dignity. Francis did not change the course of economic history, but he did effect a change of mentality with regard to those who were both rejected and aided. Everything points in this direction when we consult the Franciscan sources.

To approach this material at its loftiest point, the saint's mysticism, we must admit that in contrast to the spiritual journeys of others, Francis of Assisi does not claim to raise himself toward God by progressively making abstractions of all the experienced world and its living creatures. To merge with God, almost all mystics recommend that one detach oneself from the world; when one has thus escaped from the world, one is ready for the mystical union. Francis of Assisi proposes a journey not *from* animate creation but *in* and through it. This, at least, is what one of the great historians of Franciscan thought has stated: "It is this existential grasp of God *in* all the effects of his acting, supernatural and natural, that accounts for the lofty contemplation of Saint Francis, something that the majority of historians have not always grasped since they reduce his experience of God in the world to a procedure of analogy."[38] It is then clear—and the celebrated Canticle of Brother Sun or Canticle of the Creatures attests to it—that this man of the early thirteenth century perceived God directly in his creation, in the world, in his brothers, and made of each of them, animate or not, his brothers and sisters. Thus the poor, the lesser, the marginal become in their turn eminently sites and moments for contemplation and adoration. The poor individual was no longer one to whom you gave alms but one in whom you recognized God, one who became like a living sacrament, like the sacred itself. There is no longer any sacrality outside the fraternal bond. And the fraternal relationship finds its highest expression in the relationship with the poor.

Historians and biographers have not failed to emphasize that Francis's course of action of effective poverty had a concrete connection with the world of marginality. This was consonant with his mysticism. In fact, in a text that assuredly derives from Francis himself and that has been called his Testament we read: "This is how the Lord gave me, Brother Francis, the grace to begin to do penance. When I was still caught in sin, the sight of lepers was intolerable to me, but the Lord himself led me among them and I tended them with all my heart."[39]

The reversal in the life of the young Francis of Assisi is tied to his action of joining the poor. It seems clear that he went to a leper house. His first biographer has enhanced the event in two ways: in the first life of the saint he cherished he has Francis meet a leper on the road, and in the second life he transforms the leper into an apparition of Christ.[40] But true or embellished, this idea is of singular interest for our subject: the leper, disabled as he is, is the archetypical figure of the poor chosen by these texts. This figure is conceived as the very presence of the Lord. The disabled person is thus elevated to a status previously unknown. Spiritually, mentally, he is more than integrated: he is magnified, exalted, overvalued. The social structure foreseen for the disabled did not change. The leprosarium or hospice remained what it was. But the time is past when the disabled were seen as metaphysically and socially dangerous, were viewed as abnormalities to be situated, or were perceived as beings in need of aid. The disabled have moved to a new stage and enter into the sphere of mysticism.

I believe that we are justified in emphasizing even more the historical shift effected through Francis of Assisi by showing that his poverty, voluntary as it was, was a poverty of life *with* the poor and *like* the poor.[41] This constitutes a substantial revolution, since the monastic poverty earlier practiced in Christian communities expressed itself in quite different forms. It was a cultivated poverty, one could say, almost disinfected. The poverty of the monk, but the eventual opulence of the abbey. Ascetic poverty, but not one of sharing, unless in the form of alms to the sociological poor, those on the outside. But it is not my purpose to write a history of monastic poverty. Francis of Assisi, at the very beginning, lived among beggars, and borrowed their clothing. He was ashamed if he met anyone poorer than himself. His recent biographers all affirm: "We soon see him establishing himself with his disciples right beside the leprous and making the center for their first activity in this entrenched camp of all forms of physical and moral suffering," as a thirteenth-century source called it.[42] After the testimony of the historian who first posed the Franciscan question to which I referred earlier, here is what another well known biographer has to say: "Loving poverty is not limited to loving the poor, while seeing to it that one lacks nothing oneself; it is to make oneself poor with them . . . embracing their status and sharing their indigence. This is the form of heroism assumed by the saintliness of the blessed."[43] Claims of this kind can be multiplied. It matters little that this form of life among the poor and lepers did not last long. It also matters little that we can find much evidence, earlier than that of Francis, for the identification between the leper and Christ. The fact that the poverty of Saint Francis originally took the form of a common destiny with the wretched marks a turning point. One means of assessing how novel this was is to look at the incendiary response: Francis's father would not support his son's action (although reasonable almsgiving posed no problem) and the city of Assisi castigated him for becoming a beggar and for associating himself with those who enjoyed no status in the hierarchy. The disabled and poor had previously seen themselves as *succored;* now they found themselves glorified. The novelty is all the greater, and even the more naive, in that at the close of the twelfth century a complex of circumstances favored the beginning of revolt among the poor. The poverty movements, to which I have referred, merged with this protestation on the part of the poor. The indigent began to pose a threat and provoked outcries such as "Even the gods do not love the poor."[44] Agitation among the marginalized grew. Charitable giving ran the risk of becoming hatred and scorn. Francis chose, if we dare say use the word, this moment to go toward those on the margin and to give them a share of glory and esteem that they had previously never enjoyed. Even if he transformed nothing, he did not fail in what he had specifically set out to do: to have marginality accepted as a positive value. How much of society and of the church that was called into question by this conception can be measured by the "very clear discredit attached to poverty in the ruling circles of the church." Some of this discredit is certainly due to endless squabbling and refusals to submit to authority on the part of those who claimed succession from Francis, but there was also a basic distrust of the subversive character of the movement.

It may be remarked that in the course of this inquiry into Saint Francis I seem to have lost sight of the truly disabled, with the exception of lepers. As I said at the beginning of this chapter on the medieval period, the silence about the disabled is remarkable. Since we cannot know their exact fate, and in the absence of specific documents, I set out to understand the various mentalities and the divisions among these different mentalities. My undertaking is the reconstitution of a *cultural* history.

Social Ethics: When the Poor All Become Dangerous

This heading is intentionally ironic. After the exaltation of those who did not fit into established society, fear takes the upper hand. Beginning in the fourteenth century, we find a reining in before a danger both real and imaginary. This is the era of great epidemics, widespread dislocation and wandering, criminality. An era, in particular because of the plague, of substantial demographic and hierarchical upheaval. Great families disappeared entirely. Roving gangs sprang up. Authorities responded with repressive measures. Poverty, illness, disability, are often linked with theft, profiteering, petty criminality. Society begins to make the marginalized the object of "treatment." The almsgiving ethic now faces a difficult course; the ethic based on the indigent mystique is gone. It will prove necessary to create a framework, to reduce all the evils attributable to these situations. Too many historians of the end of the Middle Ages have written of this at length for me to presume to add anything or even summarize or synthesize. In this period too, it is problematic to distinguish the disabled from neighboring categories. I shall begin with some observations. Two studies by Bronislaw Geremek, dealing with these questions of the marginalized, are dotted with allusions to the disabled.[45] What can we learn from them? The true title of *Truands et misérables* (*Crooks and Paupers*) might be "Useless to the World, Crooks . . ." A whole operational perspective is summed up there! People on the margin have become *useless.* From useless to harmful is only a simple step. This step was taken by the legislation and judicial practice of the last quarter of the fifteenth century and the sixteenth century that "condemned anti-social behavior as a crime,"[46] a crime that could be punished by forced labor. Here is a new notion: put the marginalized to work, rehabilitate them through labor. Of course, "the ill, lame, and infirm retained a right to alms" but "their children were put in apprenticeship or in service."[47] Behind the idea of work can be seen that of *security:* institutions and group interests will seek to respond to this need. Here, too, a distinction was made between the able-bodied and those not able, but an extreme one: "When they are not able-bodied and are incapable of work, they recover their social utility, their special place in the social division of labor in that they offer the rich the possibility of acting on their charitable feelings and thus win salvation. But they remain scorned, unworthy, and deprived of all respect."[48] Under the presidency of Robert de Billy the Parliament of Rouen deliberated on the disorder created by poverty and criminality. The council was unanimous in stating "that it is necessary to distinguish and separate out the true poor, ill, feebleminded, and infirm from the vagabonds, petty thieves, and idle, all healthy and able-bodied."[49] Here we find a distinction met a bit earlier. But it should be noted that in the course of these deliberations not all the notables were in agreement. The judgment was difficult to reach. The categories of imposture are myriad. People went so far as to form groups and disguised themselves as beggars, cripples, professional mourners, paralytics, blind persons. In addition, there were "sects" of beggars among which we find the Moscarini who were maimed, the Mandragoli, the cripped in carts, the blind Abbici, the leprous and ulcer-ridden Cratersanni.[50] All of this is confused, mixed up: between the authentic and the false disabled the boundaries are not so simple. And these bands included, as well as the impaired just cited, converted Jews, pilgrims, street-singers.

These notes are of interest because they show the essentially ambiguous situation of the disabled that prevailed at the time. Clearly distinguished on the one hand and the object of traditional charity, and almost undistinguished on the other. A time of upheaval if there ever was one: the repression, forced labor, and establishment concern for security that had earlier disregarded the disabled would end up by reaching them. Like Geremek in his conclusions concerning the historical documentation on organized criminality, we may distinguish two kinds of marginality: that which challenges the social order and that, much deeper, which calls into question the organization of culture and ideology. To the former belong the robbers and rovers, to the second, the disabled or foreigners. But these two kinds of marginality are often rather confused in the general mind. Distrust, often amounting to slander, was leveled on the disabled and the ill. "It led to exclusion in two cases: that of lepers, in the Middle Ages, and that of the insane, on the threshold to the modern era. This attitude can be explained as a defensive measure against a dangerous and mysterious disease, but in the decision to isolate and sequester the sick, we also recognize the perception of their existential difference."[51]

Isolate and sequester, how was this done? Here we must refer to the evolution of the hospices and poorhouses. In the central Middle Ages, the hospice foundations were nonspecialized hostels that provided care and protection, that fed, supervised, and at times raised the needy (in particular the blind). In the fourteenth and fifteenth centuries a new trend is apparent: specialization, with the result that prostitutes, pilgrims, and the disabled are no longer mixed together. In Paris, for example, pilgrims and transients are sheltered in the Hôpital Saint-Jacques du Haut-Pas, while the foundation of Quinze-Vingts admitted only the blind. This last establishment did not intern its clients, who continued to go out and beg in the streets. The disabled and sick were directed toward the Hôtel-Dieu. What would become the hospital in the modern sense of the term accepted only these last two categories.[52] The other trend, aside from specialization, is in terms of quantity. Masses of people—even those fit for work—pressed to get in. The hospices are not yet similar to the correctional institutions they will be later. The time of the Great Internment of the classical period has not yet arrived. The practice of isolation is accentuated and tends to become more widespread. Yet there is still considerable flexibility in these arrangements at the end of the medieval period.

This, then, is what the history of marginality has to tell us.

If there were any need for additional evidence, this overview confirms the tumult of the fourteenth and fifteenth centuries. To the plagues, famines, epidemics of all kinds are to be added the wars, in the case of France, those of François I at the end of the period. In such an age, it is logical that collective attitudes and spiritual trends should be marked with pessimism. While it does not seem accurate to me to advance the thesis that the whole of the Middle Ages lived in fear of divine anger, preoccupied with ideas of sin and demonology, these themes do recur in pronounced form in times of collective calamity.

The macabre frescos, the terrifying Triumphs of Death and Last Judgments, were never so popular in ecclesiastical decoration. Sickness, but disability as well, again appears linked to sin or at least as God's punishment. Where could such a flood of misfortunes come from, if not from a judgment by God on a corrupt humanity? The popular preachers of these centuries, principally Dominicans and Franciscans, are the heralds of these ills. It will not be necessary to write at length here, since historians are in such agreement on this point. The great dignity of lepers, the disabled, sick, and, in a general way, the poor has been forgotten. They are now living reproaches by God, signs of the permission granted to the Devil. This satanic omnipresence will not begin to withdraw until the sixteenth century, when evil will be defined as a natural force, when a new medicine will be advanced as a consequence, when society will have recovered its bearings, and when the Reformation—hostile to traditional forms of charity—will make its appearance.

Having reached the end of the medieval period, I return here to what is its main root: Christianity. I have stated that the Gospels dismantle the rule of a strictly religious conception in favor of an ethical one. Let me now continue with my chosen topic. If we had to generalize—and thereby necessarily analyze—this development, I would need to write a very different book. Let readers accept my statements on the ground I have chosen. Disability, essentially conceived in a sacral relationship to the divine, experienced a kind of extradition with the arrival of the Gospels. It becomes to a much greater extent a matter of spiritual and ethical conduct. God is not absent in this view, as I have shown in the examples of Zotikos and Francis of Assisi, but his presence is very different. God sends us disease and disability as *trials* on the one hand, as *opportunities* to exercise our greatest virtue, charity, on the other, and thirdly as the *sign* of his presence. This does not entail a sacrificial attitude but puts the authenticity of our faith and our customs to the test.

But in so doing, the era of medieval Christianity never found an entirely stable position, nor an effective praxis to address disability. We have noted instability in the ways in which kinds of aberrancy and difference were situated. Their status, which was quite clear in the

classical world, and in the Jewish world even though often disadvantaged, remained very fluid in the Middle Ages. My difficulty in isolat-
ing the problem from other related questions is not simply due to the
lack of documentation but to this central fact: disability is only one of
the aspects of misery and suffering. The religious world that preceded
Christianity distinguished vigorously and sharply the aberrant character of other forms of impairment and affliction. The Christian religious world, starting with the Gospels, introduced a merger. Consequently, it could not find an original answer to the question of physical
difference; it was confused with illness, poverty, and all the unfortunate were under more or less the same sign. This situation changed
completely the fate of the disabled. Their destiny is less frightening if
we adopt an individual and humanist point of view. But otherwise,
losing their sacral function, they also lose their specificity. Not entirely
because they play at times the not inconsequential role of mocking
society. We could say, paradoxically, that people often didn't know
what to do with them except to make them springboards for charity.
The medieval attitude referred the disabled back to a more common
fate, a less extraordinary one. In so doing, it neither specified nor
treated them. On the effective level this ethical mentality is often
more passive than active, and the results may be a bit misleading.
Certainly, the good works, the foundations and institutions were not
lacking, but they, too, relegated the disabled to various forms of social
marginality. It is not incorrect to state that the Middle Ages were
hardly segregationist or elitist in the modern sense of these words.

Diversity, dissemblance, the mixed social palette were not in the
least resisted. I stated this in beginning this chapter. But the pockets
of squalor that were kept at a distance from the organization of the city
did nonetheless exist. The mentality and attitudes were variable and
ambiguous at the same time. Never truly excluded, for the disabled
were always spiritually integrated;[53] never integrated, for they were
always on the social fringes.

An inquiry into the precise situation of different disabilities on
different social strata and at each period of this long history, if such
seemed possible, would refine this perspective, but would it not call
into question the validity of my fundamental statement? I would an-

swer yet again that it is not a defense of intellectual laziness to advance the claim that the basic *principles* of division, classification, and treatment are marked by *indecision.*

These principles, attributed to Christianity, are they not the reflection of a preconceived idea of the cultural break of Christianity? It is striking that many scholars today tend to underplay the distinction between paganism and Christianity.[54] Readers will have noted, I hope, that I have not so much contrasted paganism and Christianity as the rule of religious sacrality and the system of the Gospel texts. Even if I have differentiated the Old Testament universe from that of Greco-Roman antiquity, they are both, in my opinion, similarly aligned in relation to the medieval system that derives from the New Testament.

But the question arises again: do we not give short shrift to the Middle Ages to make the era just a prolongation of the potential of the New Testament text? It is quite clear that the Middle Ages are not a simple and true reflection of Gospel principles. They are a specific historical form of Christianity that deployed its heritage in terms of a multiplicity of economic and political conditions, circumstances of climate, historical events, etc. But when matters are considered from the cultural perspective, as is my objective, in comparison with developments both before and after, the medieval period, despite undeniable decisive breaks with earlier thinking and fresh initiatives, appears, under the aegis of ethical and theological charity, to have been to a very large extent ineffective.[55]

5

The Classical Centuries: The Chill

Medicine and Philosophy

Ambroise Paré makes this distinction: "*Monsters* are beings that sur-
pass Nature, *prodigies* are things that occur in opposition to Nature,
the maimed are blind, one-eyed, hunch-backed, lame, or have six
digits on the hand or foot, or fewer than five, or have them joined
together."[1] This is a strange enumeration of deformities but an interesting classification. One might think that Ambroise Paré, writing in the
sixteenth century (1517–90), would introduce nothing new in comparison with the Middle Ages on the subject of monsters.[2] But I consider
his distinction and his vocabulary important. That I begin this new
period with reference to a physician is an indication of my position. If
medieval culture put itself under the sign of the Christian ethic, the
era that now opens will distance itself from it in profound ways. This
does not signify that it will be an age of medicalization. I simply want
to say, at the beginning, that the priest, monk, or friar is no longer our
means of access to the new cultural era.

Let us follow for a moment the progress of medicine in the century of Paré. "The father of modern surgery recognizes that mental
illness has a material cause, because it can be transmitted by heredity."[3] The interest of Paré's statement does not lie in its random character in the eyes of present-day science. But by introducing heredity,
Paré eliminated the theory of demonology. His Swiss contemporary,
Félix Plater, from the same medical perspective, protested against the
punishment inflicted on the mentally ill. At the end of the century, the
Italian, Gazoni, proposed that the insane be admitted to hospitals. In

parallel fashion and especially because of the appearance of syphilis, the idea of contagion was born. The great plagues had not provoked reflection on the natural propagation of epidemics. The sixteenth century began to rid itself of the idea of divine justice in favor of that of contagion, including as an underlying "watermark," in Sendrail's image, the idea of microbic infection. Certainly the intellectual climate has changed since the terrors at the close of the Middle Ages, even if epidemics would continue for several more centuries. These first thoughts about contagion will lead to inoculation and vaccination at the end of the eighteenth century (as observed by Jenner in 1796).

My purpose here is not to retrace the history of medicine. The birth of psychiatric thought and the birth of medicine based on the observation of natural processes are two examples that demonstrate that a new system of thought has been inaugurated.

To follow the development of this system we have the advantage, as concerns "madness," of the work of Foucault, which continues to be an obligatory point of reference. The philosophical initiative that underlies Foucault's works and in particular his *Histoire de la folie à l'âge classique* (*History of Madness in the Classical Age*) has been much discussed. It is not my aim to engage in this debate at the present time. Additionally, his methodology, in particular his division into periods, has also been questioned.[4] For my part, I am content to leave Foucault's work, with its impressive beauty and its penetrating vision of *le grand enfermement*, "the Great Confinement," without further comment. Mental illness and the repressive treatment it received in the classical period will be discussed only in passing. There is no need to redo something that, for the present, remains so well done.

But Foucault has left a whole continent unexplored: physical disability.

In the Middle Ages, we have seen, people spoke lightly of monsters and monstrosity without having seen them. It was an imaginary world. Even in the case of major human deformities, people recounted incidents that were never verified. And this lore was passed on for generations. Then medical thought of a more scientific kind makes its appearance. Like Paré, it breaks with the idea of demonic visitation and curses in order to seek the origins of deformity via the causal categories established by Aristotle. Several different causes were entertained, for example, the imaginings of the mother. A child's deformity could result, they thought (and people would continue to think for a very long time), from images, nightmares, perceptions experienced by the mother. However unrefined such a conception of causality may have been, it did show that thinkers were looking to a natural sequence of events and no longer to a moral one.

But the true situation was not quite so simple, and lengthy discussions would be held between 1670 and 1745,[5] linked to the question of heredity and the preexistence of "germs" (in the sense of seed). To state the situation briefly, two great perspectives stood in contrast. Some would claim that aberration comes from God and is part of creation by reason of a superior normality. God is the direct author of laws, and himself gives to nature its natural character (*natura naturans*). The germs of everything have been placed by God in the world. Thus the aberrant germs are as ordained as any others and come from his wisdom. Aberrations and deformities are equally rational: in their structure they are just as functional as normal organisms and, moreover, they are part of that immense intelligence of the world that is beyond our ken. Here we can recognize the influence of Saint Augustine in part, although the emphasis has been somewhat shifted. In fact, it is the internal reasonableness of the malformation that is at the focal point. In addition, there is no longer talk of reported instances, but existing malformations are presented in various scholarly circles where efforts are made to account for them. Among the thinkers of the time we find representatives of Jansenism such as Arnauld or Régis.[6] From this perspective the malformed are such only for us, not in relation to nature, in which the will of God and his unfathomable possibilities are manifest. But this meant denying the very idea of *aberrance*. As Régis says, reality may be extraordinary, but it is not irregular, and it is not an error. In 1706 the physician Duverney presented before the French Academy the case of two infants united at the pelvis, born in Vitry on September 20 of that year: "The 'creator's mechanics' is praised for its richness at the expense of its order, and is no more than the ingeniousness of a craftsman who creates an original device."[7]

A second current of thought held that anomalies do not originate with the Creator but are due to accidents that occur during the development of the germ. Perfect germ perhaps, but faulty development. This current of thought strives in the direction of empirical observation and away from theology, even though all thinkers of the time had to face the problem of creation by God. But for the proponents of this second position, there was a problem concerning human knowledge. God may have made things perfectly, but we can know them. If we can know them, one should not have recourse to mystifying explanations. A philosopher such as Malebranche assumes this viewpoint. The so-called rationality of Duverney was scarcely tenable in the long run. Let us then accept the idea that the development of germs may be aberrant and let us look for the explanation in a series of natural causes. The weakness of this school of thought lies in the fact that it had at its disposal only mechanical causes: constriction of the uterus, crushing of the germ. It was the scholar Winslow who brilliantly discredited this theory of crushed germs in his confrontation with a partisan of the second perspective, Lémery, who insisted on claiming that monstrosity is monstrosity. Lémery died before Winslow, who went on to shade his own position by admitting the possibility of accidents: "The theory of accidents could not satisfactorily explain certain indisputable facts; to make God immediately responsible for monsters is repugnant to reason. To exit from this dilemma we must renounce the idea of the pre-existence of germs, that is, of the passivity of nature."[8]

As it happened, the confrontation was to prove sterile in the sense that it was no more than a conflict between two intellectual positions that had an identical starting point. Thinkers had to free themselves of the idea that nature was a mechanism elaborated by God and was incapable of forming a living being on its own. A new idea of nature and of life had to be conceived.

But for me what is valuable in this debate is that thinkers tried to account for what they observed, even at the cost of theological conceptions, and that the discussions were conducted within the Academies. This approach is different from that of the Middle Ages.

Although I shall not return in the following to the question of monstrosity, it should be noted that the discussion does not stop with post-Cartesian polemics. But in its essentials it abandons its fundamental concern with functional and evolutionary ideas of the living. We may cite as example the great elucidation made by Jules Guérin in the nineteenth century.[9] We see a clear conceptual distinction between deformity and monstrosity, but, at the same time, through a graduated causal sequence, a claim for a link between monstrosity and the deformity that accompanies it to "one and the same causal order, cerebrospinal disorders" (527). Guérin eliminates as determining causes such factors as the imaginings of the mother, the influence of moral impairment, heredity, the age of the parents, social station, direct body pressure, attempts at abortion, etc., as well as all the other earlier theories that I have cited. His single explanation is the effect of lesions, a theory that he will advance from 1840 to 1880 (708 ff.).

Thus we are led, on the level of ideas, to the prelude to the great undertaking of the Encyclopedia and the intellectual expansion of the Enlightenment. But before advancing, it will be rewarding to have a look at the social praxis of the sixteenth and seventeenth centuries. The learned world of the time did indeed take up the problem of aberrance and monstrosity, but elsewhere, in real life, there was the world of the disabled. Are we not still in the presence of a classification that neatly separates the universe of congenital *deformity* from that of inherent or acquired *disability?*

This can be established for the preceding periods, and the difference is often a clear one. In one way or another, however, the two questions abut another and merge. In the Middle Ages, for example, the monster is primarily an imaginary complex of features, but the characteristics ascribed to disability are also borrowed from monstrosity, and there is the admixture of social marginalization. In antiquity deformity, even that not of a monstrous nature, is an aberration that is just as intolerable, but antiquity separated *disability at birth* from all other impairments. What is the situation during the great centuries of science, philosophy, and literature?

Charity and Internment

While this long polemic on monstrosity was running its course, what was being done for those who, even if not monstrous, were nonetheless referred to monstrosity by their disability? It seems as though there were attempts to resolve both questions at once, the problem of monstrosity and that of the disabled. But were these not two incommensurable quantities? It is difficult to say. Perhaps one could advance the thesis that to the extent that rationalism and its intellectual rigor informed all efforts at understanding in the seventeenth century, in particular at understanding the monster, all forms of non-conformity had to be similarly situated, given an assigned place. For there is one common thing shared by the two currents of thought that debated monstrosity: reason would be able to situate it exactly in the scheme of things, either in order to refer it to a higher reason, that of God, or in order to grasp the processes that produce it. Situating monstrosity on the intellectual level is perhaps not so far removed from the social space that is assigned to all marginality. This space, under the command of reason, is the confines of the hospital. And thus we rejoin Foucault.

For this reason and for others as well, we shall have to go back and trace the concrete treatment of disability. Let us return to the very beginning of the Great Century, the seventeenth century in France. Testimony is discouragingly spare. If we think, for example, of the life and work of Vincent de Paul, who incarnated and symbolized charity in the first half of the century, we scarcely meet the disabled at all.[10] Vincent de Paul concerned himself with misery of all kinds: the situation of foundlings, convicts, prisoners, the sick, aged, prostitutes, beggars, but we never see him with the disabled, unless by chance, if some of the indigent were also maimed. There was no specialized institutional apparatus until the foundation of the Hôtel des Invalides hospital by Louis XIV. I shall return to this. We must then conclude that the disabled did not constitute a serious social problem. At the close of the Middle Ages they continued to form part of the poor in general, unless they were completely hidden within the family home, or even if they were not smothered, as infants, in the parents' bed.[11] From this point of view it is not without interest to scrutinize the celebrated charity of the seventeenth century, which was intended to encompass the disabled.

Everyone wholeheartedly agrees with Foucault that this century, particularly through the establishment of the Hôpital Général in

1656, unfolded under the sign of promoting the rule of (social) order and thus with the practice of interning the poor and the insane. And in this classical period "all power was called charitable," since the whole deployment of charity contributed, in fact if not in intention, to the exercise of political power with a view to circumscribing aberrance formally.[12] Is this true of Vincent de Paul? One of his biographers of the last century[13] began by showing his renewal of ties with the first Christian generations, before Constantine and the hospice foundations, through charity at home, close to the individual poor. His recommendations were always to visit the poor, and les Filles de la Charité (the Daughters of Charity) began in this spirit. Having said this, the biographer goes on to claim that the hospice was, in the seventeenth century, the only possible form of charity. I seem to see in this paradox more than simple inattention on the part of Arthur Loth or a simple evolution in the life of Vincent. It is the very ambivalence of charity as it was conceived and positioned in the seventeenth century that is called into question here. Vincent de Paul, faced with the spread of squalor after the religious wars (which was widely recognized) and with the destruction of the network of hospices that had been run by the church, invents a form of charity made up of an emotional evangelism, a will to succor and educate, and the intention to restore the kingdom of France to health. These three objectives are almost always united in his efforts. The works that he established—the seventeenth century is the age of public works—are marked by these elements in balance. The indigent have an "eminent dignity," according to Bossuet, and must be approached as one would Jesus Christ himself, but the poor must accept instruction (particularly in matters of religion), and people must submit to the order of the king, God's lieutenant.

It is symptomatic that Vincent de Paul always wanted multifunctional Filles de la Charité or Prêtres de la Mission (Priests of the Mission) in the institutions that housed the assistance activity, the "little school," and the official chaplaincy or almshouse. But we also see that these components, which Vincent saw united, could also become autonomous. This is the case of la Compagnie du Saint Sacrement (the Company of the Holy Sacrament; an *Opus Dei* before its time?), which Vincent de Paul distrusted. It was a clique of the devout that served public order more than evangelical charity, and it came to occupy a position that the king, Louis XIV, did not appreciate. And for his part, too, Vincent de Paul did not view the Hôpital Général favorably, because it resembled a policing operation and neglected the misery out in the provinces. He did not introduce religious sisters into the hospitals until fairly late;[14] all his life he remained attached to individualized aid. But despite all that, he did institutionalize charity, ran with a firm hand his home for the elderly, la Maison du Nom de Jésus (the Home of the Name of Jesus), where artisans' work was to be performed,[15] and gathered indigent poor behind walls. He insisted throughout his life on the instruction of the poor. Here he was not without influence on the complex relationship between the elite, whom this favored, and the lower classes. The fate of the poor, although alleviated, was not transformed, and Bourdaloue could write, "The poor were necessary so that there might be subordination and order in human society."[16]

Saint Vincent de Paul should not simply be associated with the Great Confinement, which inaugurates a new phase of administrative repression in the treatment of the poor. The principal accomplishment of Vincent de Paul predates the fateful year of 1656 that saw the creation of the notorious "general hospitals" (*hôpitaux généraux*). But, on the other hand, it would not be honest to exculpate Vincent de Paul entirely from this movement toward internment. This institutionalization, whatever its apostolic character, was relative and fairly mild in houses that he founded but nonetheless entailed concentrating people with a view to establishing order. Vincent de Paul was certainly a pastor in the fundamental sense of the word, and his objective was the Christianization of the poor. The concrete exercise of charity was the criterion, the means to effect this conversion; even more, the apostolic ministry merged with the charitable ministry. But the ministry was also caught in undeniable cultural constraints. The first constraint originated in the Counter-Reformation. Vincent de Paul belonged to the tradition of the Council of Trent. Even if it is difficult to say that charitable works declined because of doctrinal reform concerning the relationship between faith and works,[17] Vincent de Paul supported this practice of works of mercy to counterbalance reformist ideas. In addition, in the second half of the sixteenth century, when Vincent de Paul was born, a Catholic doctrine of charity had also seen the light of day. Juan-Luis Vives, a scholarly theologian, while leaving the funding of charity to private alms-giving, promoted obligatory work for the poor, prison for vagabonds, internment (without harsh treatment) of the insane. The same doctrine is found advanced by Dominic Soto, with a tendency toward supporting charitable works from public funds.[18] Charity, of which Vincent de Paul is the leading exponent, is to be located on a vector of control, containment, and order. It is not inconsistent with the Hôpital Général.

But did the disabled escape the Hôpital Général or not? We should recall that the Hôpital Général, the policing agent for the poor, permitted the continuation of all the earlier hospices, the Hôtels-Dieu. And in these hospitals, we find sections reserved for the infirm, such as in the celebrated Apostolic Hospital of Saint Michael in Rome. There were even specialized institutions, such as the Hôpital des Incurables (Hospital for the Incurable) in Paris.[19] Saint Vincent de Paul, in a lecture to Les Filles de la Charité, enjoined them to exclude from their houses those with edema (dropsy), the lame and one-handed, because the Incurables was there for them.[20] Without being incarcerated, a repressive fashion in the Hôpital Général, the disabled did tend to be interned. They were sequestered, we must insist, in a different way than in the hospices of the Middle Ages: not so much in order to care and treat them better medically than during the Middle Ages but in order to concentrate their numbers. Whether a specialized concentration or not, there was a clear delimitation of territory, something that the Middle Ages had not attempted for comparable reasons.

The most striking example of delimitated space for the disabled is the creation of the Hôtel des Invalides, a facility for wounded and disabled veterans, whose founding edict was signed at Versailles in 1674 by Louis XIV. Before the projects that culminated in the Invalides and during the medieval period, disabled ex-soldiers were billeted (as oblates or lay brothers) in abbeys that were to maintain them.[21] The oblates were pensioned. With the onset of the religious wars, their number grew, and the abbeys were ruined. Moreover, this administrative practice tended to fall into disuse because many abbots opposed it, and veterans with rights profited by the situation and had themselves received several times over as lay brothers at different houses. Faced with these difficulties, Henri IV formally approved an establishment that already existed on rue Lourcine in Paris. This was La Maison de la Charité Chrétienne (the House of Christian Charity), from which pensioners had the right to obtain a uniform. After the assassination of Henri IV, the situation reverted to what it had been earlier. Disabled veterans were sent home with a modest sum of money. During the reign of Louis XIII one man, Charmot, made this his crusade. In 1633, the king finally set up a commune as a chivalric order (la Commanderie Saint-Louis) and had a building erected on the site of the castle of Bicêtre. He thought to finance the operation by taxing the abbeys, which were no longer fulfilling their former role. But then came the hostility of the clergy, the disorder of the Fronde, the death of Louis XIII, and the project was deferred. Several other solutions were advanced. In 1644 an ordinance was passed to collect up the crippled veterans who were begging and send them to military posts on the borders of France. The maimed ex-soldiers were roused to action, and it proved necessary to forbid giving them alms. In 1670 Louis XIV decided to put up a domiciliary (*hôtel*) and returned to the idea of a fund composed of the former pensions that the abbeys were no longer paying their pensioners. Then, in 1674, came the Edict of Versailles and the definitive establishment, more or less on the present-day site of the Invalides in Paris. Since not all the needy were in Paris and many disabled soldiers rejected the idea of a sedentary life (and a very regulated one, as in a convent), detached companies of disabled veterans were also created, again in frontier locations. In 1702 there were sixty-one companies of this nature. These soldiers, still formally in the army, were not all disabled to the same degree, or even all disabled. They were a mixture of veterans and the invalided out. The assignment to the residence in Paris or to one of the distant posts was imposed by the authorities and was not a free choice.[22]

The later history of the Invalides need not concern us here. Let us simply say that in the eighteenth century there were difficulties with money . . . and with discipline. In 1724 an ordinance reestablished order by making entry into the Invalides a reward based on merit. Choiseul increased the number of pensions in 1764 so that the war wounded would stay home. The Convention would make some modifications but left the essentials in place.

This institution and health service facility was intended to check delinquency, but also to avoid the mistakes of the Hôpital Général.[23] Louis XIV wanted to make the Invalides a model infirmary and long-term care facility, rather on the pattern of the houses of Vincent de Paul: good hygiene, heating, surgery, a regulated atmosphere but alleviated by the presence of the "gray sisters" (the Filles de la Charité). The surgical ward of the Invalides, under the two Morands, father and son, would become famous and trend-setting. This did not hide the fact that internment persisted. Within the walls the veterans worked. Louvois would create real manufacturing units that produced shoes and tapestries, and cut out material for clothing. In 1683 the overseer for the shops would be a disabled veteran who had worked his way up from the floor, Jean Gautier.[24]

Concentrated, interned, and transformed into productive workers—this is what the Great Century and its great king introduced for disabled ex-soldiers. This same king would export the formula as far as Canada when he granted subsidies to a certain François Charron (whose name is today borne by an institution for the disabled in Quebec) in order to set up workshops for the disabled in this overseas province.

The poor were not to be idle. This concern, which would become a major one and even take root among the disabled themselves, was completely absent during the medieval period. The workshops or charity shops—such organized charity would be the type that predominated—would become very numerous. We know how zealously Turgot, in the eighteenth century, built on the ideas of Louis XIV. But in 1791 the shops would be closed down. Were the disabled themselves involved? Clearly, the shops had not been created for them, but for the poor. And it is equally true that we have no firm evidence of the presence of the disabled in the shops. But we sense the overall policy environment and this large-scale social action with regard to the poor would also affect the impaired and the powerless.[25]

Biology and Humanism

Earlier we followed the debate of the seventeenth century concerning monstrosity. This preoccupation seems to withdraw a bit during the Age of Enlightenment. Maupertuis, for example, just mentions the disagreement between Lémery and Winslow without adding a personal opinion. This can be understood against the background of what Jacques Roger calls skepticism, whether it be conventionally religious, deist, or atheist: we must return to the real but give up trying to dominate it by the intelligence. In the fashion of insects—which were of great interest to the eighteenth century—anomalies are curiosities to be inventoried but are not susceptible to explanation.

The baton will, however, be taken up by Diderot in his famous "Letter on the blind for the use of the sighted." The context of this letter is of interest for my subject. It introduces Nicholas Saunderson, who actually existed. Blind and a professor of mathematics at Cambridge, he was the first to invent a method for the blind to learn arithmetic. The method was reinvented by Henry Moves, blind as well and a lecturer in chemistry in Edinburgh.[26] These first methods would be pursued at the very close of the eighteenth century and perfected for the instruction of the blind. In Germany and Austria Christian Nielsen and J.-L. Weissemburg developed a writing system. In France, there was the work of Valentin Haüy, and in Scotland, again, the writings of Thomas Blacklock, in particular an important article in the *Encyclopedia Britannica*. In short, there was a completely new concern: for *education* and the *rehabilitation of the disabled.* But for a century still, the blind would constitute an exception, at least as concerns apprenticeship and retraining, for in the case of the poor and aberrant the training initiatives would be of a moral nature. The idea, however, of formally organizing the disabled and returning them to the level of others makes its entry into history, along with ideas for appropriate technologies and specialized institutions.[27] But let us return to Diderot and his "Letter on the blind," which won him a stay at the Vincennes prison. What strikes the reader most on the superficial level is the attention accorded to the psychology of the blind and thus also to the rehabilitation of these physically impaired.

After Diderot interest will be great across all of Europe. The potential, the intellectual, artistic, literary, and scientific possibilities, of the blind will be highlighted. This will be done in stages, for the pioneers whom I have mentioned often emphasized one particular capacity of the blind in a particular way, as if there were some domains reserved for their talents and others forbidden to just that disability. There was a time when the blind were thought particularly suited for music. But the interest of Diderot's text is not limited to the psychology of the vision impaired. With his work the author changes the problematics of monstrosity and—even more generally—the problematics of biological transmission. Saunderson is a monster: "Look at me closely, Mr. Holmes, I have no eyes. What have we done to God, you and I, the one in order to have these organs, the other to be deprived of them?" (43). The question of God's role in the generation of species permits Diderot to leave his earlier deism for a resigned atheism, as Roger says. The species, like the monsters who never form a species, are due to chance, where the one that adapts persists and the one that fails to adapt disappears. Diderot is not at all a transformationalist before his time, because he would then be defending an order and a teleology by citing the emergence and evolution of species. *But there is no longer a divine order.* Thus Diderot rejoins Buffon when the latter states that the universe is not an ordered creation but a "world of relative and non-relative beings, an infinity of harmonious and opposing combinations, and destruction and renewal in perpetuity."[28]

I shall not address the exact conceptions of Diderot as these relate to the history of the life sciences. What is important for me is that the "Letter on the blind," abandoning the debates of the preceding century, establishes the lines of inquiry of the biological sciences, and the idea that the genesis of life is to be described and understood without recourse to such conceptions as preexistent germs. Diderot's text inaugurates the period when aberrancy, monstrosity, diminished faculties, and deformity will be addressed as simple impairments. They will be understood from within, subjectively. Finally, they begin to be the objects of remedial treatment. The new ground broken by Diderot's letter is considerable, even if it is to be seen as a continuation from the intellectual break of the sixteenth century, which was even more decisive.

Along with Diderot's statement and the possibilities that it opens, internment was no less a reality, especially for the mentally ill whose conditions were terrible. Imprisoned, or more accurately caged and chained, they were kept with vagabonds and criminals, even exhibited like animals in a zoo. A certain number of the physically disabled were also in this situation. The actual praxis of the period must never be forgotten, even if our concern here is with changes in perspective.

But, even on the level of praxis, a change was in the offing. A sharper scientific focus (in particular as concerns transmission, species, heredity), the more effective medical treatment of many afflictions, the will no longer to accept as destiny what is made in society and can be modified by it—all this favored what we might call a humanization of the lot of the aberrant, a willingness to address these situations through appropriate technology. Pinel arrives on the scene, and will reform the hospital and create a new space, the asylum. We are witness to the emergence of a new power, medical power, and to the nearly totalitarian ambition of this power. The year 1770 may serve as reference point for this development—incredible in its effects, since it will dominate the two following centuries, that is, until the present day. In 1770 physicians paid by the royal administration begin to spread across the French countryside. This is the realization of the medical profession's great dream to care for the ill and in so doing to become the adjudicators of a social norm that is defined on the basis of norms of life and of health. At the close of the eighteenth century this dream of medical power, which had the mandate to serve, or even to dominate, political power, was effectively made reality.[29] The dream will be thwarted by the Napoléon's establishment of a centralized administration. But the fact remains that the power of medicine, in particular through the family physician on the one hand and through the uncontested dominance of the new institution of the asylum on the other, would become definitively installed by the close of the eighteenth century. In the psychiatric sphere social control will be applied to every appearance of abnormality through the coercive medium of the hospital for the insane. In the family sphere the general practitioner will become a kind of counselor, a new kind of priest. Within administrations themselves there will be a need for expertise and medical opinions. "Without recourse to medicine, no life is possible,"[30] and thus no social life either. Jean-Pierre Peter is right when he states, "The pronounced fervor of physicians to contain society in its entirety in order to bring it to live according to the norm: with very differing general conditions for its realization, public pronouncements, formal arrangements, this is what inscribes this earlier age and today's in one and the same perspective" (183 f.). This was permitted, at least in part, by the "biologization" of thought during the Age of Enlightenment. The great scientific and medical works, oriented toward life and its riches—in contrast to the seventeenth century and its focus on physics—had as a consequence that medicine and the medical profession were brought to the front rank of society. If the insane and developmentally retarded are henceforth entirely under the control of the medical establishment,[31] is this equally true of the physically disabled?

I said earlier that I would not recall the works of Foucault. We should remember, however, that the seventeenth century was the period of the Great Confinement in the Hôpital Général, with all categories thrown together. The goal of this massive internment was to avoid the *danger* that different marginalities represented. Otherwise, as far as madness was concerned, it was a matter of showing that reason and unreason had nothing in common and thus to have a certain kind of reason win out. We know that the relationship between reason and unreason is once again being modified in our century, in particular following the emergence of the theories of Freud.

The Great Confinement of the classical age was transformed under the influence of eighteenth-century ideas with the arrival of Pinel at the Bicêtre facility (1793) and with the career of this physician. The hodgepodge of the Hôpital Général will come to an end but only to be replaced by the asylum, which will be well organized and specialized. Initially, this new internment will not be particularly medicalized in the therapeutic sense of the word but will, above all else, serve the ends of social control through a kind of moral oversight. Real medicalization will come only at the end of the nineteenth century. These comments give but a rough impression of the quite remarkable and detailed book by Robert Castel, to which I refer readers.

Assistance and Restoration

Unlike those called insane, many of the disabled could not be assimilated to the sick. This is apparent at numerous moments in history: impairment and reduced mental ability are clearly separated from disability or deformity. Today a complete juncture has been effected. But the incurable nature of a number of disabilities, tied to the trainable potential of those subject to them, caused disability to follow a different course in the nineteenth century than either physical illness or psychological illness. The disabled person, particularly the physically disabled one, starts to take on specific contours, well distinguished from monstrosity, sickness, and madness. A kind of remediation has begun, but not through incarceration or therapy or even through a more or less sacral valorization.

Let us begin by describing the empirical situation. Two kinds of cases deserve comment: deaf-mutes and the blind. It should be noted that these two conditions had the benefit of a certain tradition. For the deaf and mute the Benedictine Pedro Ponce de León, who died in 1584, seems to have been the first to begin refining a method of communication and instruction. He will be followed by men such as Juan Pablo Bonet, also a Spaniard, John Wallis in England (1660), Jean Conrad Amman in Switzerland (1724), Petro de Castro in Italy, and above all the celebrated abbé de l'Épée in Paris in the eighteenth century. It was the last-named who most worked for the introduction and use of sign language, while others made greater use of drawings and lip-reading. The abbé de l'Épée (1712–89) would live to see his work carried forward, and his accomplishment remains until the present day. The first German institution stimulated by the abbé de l'Épée's ideas opened in 1778.

The idea of remedial training or rehabilitation for the disabled was then not new, but it put down solid roots, for some categories at least, at the end of the Age of Enlightenment, as evidenced by the concern for the blind, led by the great pioneer Valentin Haüy (1745–1822). Although contemporaries, the abbé de l'Épée and Valentin Haüy were not at all associated, but they were engaged in the same struggle: through the intervention of appropriate techniques, people with sensory disability could gain access to an intellectual, artistic, professional life.

It is not part of the purpose of this book to give a biography of these two precursors.[32] Like all founders, they focused on a single concept of great power, simple in its realization: the *education* (in its broadest sense) of those who were thought afflicted with radical incapacity and who were classified in a kind of subhuman category. They were also able to convince others, upsetting the whole social construction of the psychology and mental faculties of persons with sensory deficiencies. But above all, they created specialized institutions, intended to offset the objective obstacles that hindered access to a personal and social life. It was no longer a question of simply gathering the disabled together, or even of putting them to work as less than able-bodied. The objective was rather to provide entry to the common cultural and social heritage of their fellow citizens. This mission was assumed by particular, specialized institutions. At the same time as these innovators rehabilitated and educated the disabled, they institutionalized them as well. In these establishments, in addition to the great sense of solidarity that would reign there and the powerful stimulus the disabled would exert on one another, some very significant work was to be accomplished. This was the invention of an alphabet of raised dots for the blind, to which Louis Braille, a student at the institution founded by V. Haüy, would give his name.[33] Much later came a remarkable synthesis on the psychology of the blind.[34] But enough of these examples, which cannot be exhaustive.

These institutions, however fruitful they were and are, remained institutions. They are the forerunners in many respects of what would become in our century the almost single formula for persons afflicted with malformations, inherent or acquired. The governing ideas of today's rehabilitation are already present in the institutions of V. Haüy and the abbé de l'Épée: the claim that the disabled can tap into the same assets as the able-bodied; the invention of techniques and pedagogies to achieve these goals; the foundation of specialized institutions to make this all possible. From this came the thought that there should only be customized institutions that were geared to dealing with the particular situation of their clientele. But the difference between this conception and that of our own era—and this will turn out to be a considerable rupture—is that Valentin Haüy and others had no pretension to integrate the disabled into ordinary life and in particular into ordinary work.

Another great advocate of the blind, Maurice de la Sizeranne (1857–1924), the successor to Haüy in the following century, states that the light of the blind is hard work.[35] In 1893 he organized a purse workshop, which would be followed by others. In this founder of the Valentin Haüy Association, propagator of the Braille method, which was still the object of controversy, and a very cultivated man, we already find in part what would become the great theme of the twentieth century. Maurice de Sizeranne, particularly in *Trente ans d'études et de propagande en faveur des aveugles* (*Thirty Years of Studies and Propaganda on Behalf of the Blind* [1893]), proves himself both a traditionalist and an innovator. He distrusted institutionalization, the status of which he nonetheless contributed to strengthen, because of its cold and dangerous character. This is why—and here he is simply reflective of his period—he wanted his association to be a family ("from the cradle to the grave") in terms of both atmosphere and size. He was ill disposed toward adopting for the blind the schools for the sighted (*Note sur les aveugles*, 1893, 18) but otherwise did not want the institution to uproot the blind person from life of the family kind.

The examples of the blind and the deaf put us on a route toward the twentieth century, with the themes of rehabilitation and specialized institutions. But training, especially in the form of conventional schooling, which was a principal goal of these foundations, was still very far from what we, today, would call reintegration and redeployment. Then it was a matter of drawing impaired persons out of inactivity and lack of culture, the results of prejudice concerning their capacity. The implications are more humanist and moral than social. The disabled are to be "raised up," restored. This restoration will shortly begin to serve the bourgeois revolution, which will set up its own customs and its own constraints as a general model: the proletariat worker and every poor person with him will become the object of charitable attention in order to get him to accept (if possible) the ways of the dominant group. This educational recovery will be accompanied by a sociological recovery. The ideas of the abbé de l'Épée and of Valentin Haüy are not those of the paternalistic charity that was prominent in the nineteenth century; they belong to the Age of Enlightenment. But they also nurtured bourgeois moralism because they were ideas of education and of remediation on the cultural level.

Are these two instances of people with sensory disability isolated? In France, and from the point of view of institutions, the answer is yes. We do not find other, parallel efforts, either public or private, for other impairments during the nineteenth century.[36] This is not the case everywhere, as we shall see. We must initially bear in mind that it is only very recently that certain afflictions were described medically and became objects of attention. Earlier those subjects who might have been afflicted by them did not survive. This is the case of myopathy, for example, or of certain kidney ailments. Some other disabilities, such as cerebral palsy, were confused with developmental retardation, since they had been neither explained nor made the object of therapy. In our eyes today, these are false cases of developmental retardation, ones where effects were considered causes. These remarks, whatever their importance, beg the question: motor disabilities existed, along with intellectual deficiencies. What was done about them? For these malformations or disabilities, two principal solutions were attempted in the nineteenth century.

The family circle tried to retain and raise impaired children as best it could. But in the nineteenth century the family was transformed, as we all know since the vogue of family studies. The family became restricted and nuclear, based on the married couple and on emotions of love, emotions of which a great deal would be demanded in the private sphere. But the family, which in our century has become incapable of functioning as a supporting locus for disability, began by being highly valued (Maurice de la Sizeranne was a good witness). "Familialism" is one of the distinguishing features of the nineteenth century. For a certain time the family (let us, for the sake of convention, take the middle-class model generated by industrial society) assumed missions, in particular with regard to the child, whose importance would greatly increase. During this period the disabled person occasionally finds a place and a haven within the family. But this is not the general case, for the disabled person is often indigent and a burden.

When the family was lacking, there was a second set of solutions: the Hôpital Général or the traditional Hôtel-Dieu or the provincial hospice. More and more services were being made available for the incurably ill and impaired, where elderly bedridden persons were side by side with young cripples and the mentally impaired of all kinds. The asylum, which has been so studied with regard to insanity, set a trend. It was not an environment of care, but an internment, a stockade that scarcely guaranteed more than survival but allowed society to hide and regulate human misery. The covering veil was at times so thick that exhibiting disability, and/or exploiting it, became more frequent in the nineteenth century than previously. Admittedly, voyeurism in this domain is of long standing, but the fairs and public holiday celebrations were never so rife with monstrosities on exhibit or with disabled persons on tour. Vincent de Paul, on occasion, did save children who had been mutilated in order to make beggars of them or simply children who had a profitable disability. But in the nineteenth century the concern for sordid reality grew, including its components of curiosity and exploitation. I would not make the exploitation of deficiency through beggary a characteristic of one culture or another, since it is to be found to a certain extent everywhere. As unfortunate and detestable as they are, such practices are never fundamental to a society.

I must be emphatic on this point. The nineteenth century, particularly in France but in Europe generally, will be dominated by aid in the form of reclusion, alongside the concern for rehabilitation. To flesh out the details of this development, we must return to the Revolution.

It should be said at the outset that the ideas of the Revolution scarcely lasted longer than the Revolution itself. More than a century would pass before certain arrangements that had been forged in the fire of the various revolutionary assemblies would be taken up again.

The Constituent Assembly had set up a Committee on Beggary whose principles were as follows: *assistance is a social duty*[37] (this refrain will be repeated in all reports to the assemblies); *making provisions for public assistance* is a necessity in order to reduce incapacity; *private benevolence* should be encouraged. From these principles, the committee gave its preference to *help in the home;* its fourth report stated: "Indeed, it is through mutual care that the spirit of the family is conserved, that natural bonds are strengthened, that kindness is cultivated, and that habits are improved."[38] Institutionalization was not excluded by the revolutionaries, who anticipated an asylum reserved for the aged and the disabled in every department of France and another in every city of more than 100,000 inhabitants. As concerns the disabled in particular, assistance was to be provided to them after age sixty; they were to be admitted to institutions only after age seventy (except in the case of severe disability).[39]

Thus, if the Constituent Assembly did not exclude hospitalization of the disabled—at the same time as it established the *crimes* of begging and vagrancy—emphasis was nonetheless on assistance and not on exclusion and repression. Admittedly, one can see in these measures of the Constituent Assembly—as some have done in the case of the mentally ill[40]—primarily a logic to effect social control: aid to the poor is required so that there may no longer be an excuse for begging, vagrancy, parasitism. One can also show that on the basis of this logic, medicine will be swallowed up in the "legality" of which the Revolution was so fond and would become the regulatory device for aberrancy, in a mixture of "compassion and science," of "benevolence and authority."[41] The transfer of social responsibility (and thereby policing responsibility) to medicine was complete in the case of mental aberrancy but much less so for physical impairment. We can, however, agree that, through the preferential status accorded the hospital, these shifts in power in the nineteenth century were also evident in the case of the disabled. But not at the time of the Constituent Assembly. The Convention will adopt the same basic measures, although with a different vocabulary: assistance is a justified national expense, but begging is a crime; if one is able-bodied, one should work, if one is disabled, one will be helped. The Convention would pass much legislation dealing with the problem but would accomplish little. Aiming too high resulted in only modest gains, because of the abusive potential of the spirit of centralization and nationalization. The Directory insisted on assistance in the home, while also reviving a certain operational role for the hospitals,[42] with offices of community welfare. Through this reorganization of local aid and the reconstitution of hospital resources, public assistance enters a new phase: it becomes optional (and no longer a national duty) and ultimately evolved into what would characterize the nineteenth century: very strictly charitable assistance. It is true that in 1848 an effort would be made to return to the spirit of the Revolution, but this would be only a short episode. It is no longer a matter of national obligation, and legislators would wait until 1905 before again addressing the rights of the disabled. There remains private benevolence, which would generate such organizations as the Society of Saint Vincent de Paul, which will not be concerned with the disabled except as they join in the larger destiny of all the indigent. This benevolence took the form of overnight hostels, heated open shelters, soup kitchens, dispensaries, assisted housing. These charitable works developed at random, with attendant waste and inevitable duplication. In 1890 the Central Office of Charitable Works was created, but this did not provide a solution on the scale of the problem. This is why—and here we return to public assistance—help in the form of hospitalization became the principal solution, even if aid at home continued, administered through the local welfare offices. In 1905 there were 69,619 public beds designated for the aged, disabled, and incurable.

In principle the aged and incurable went to the hospices and the sick to the hospitals. But in actual fact, the mixture of categories was considerable and the disabled are found everywhere: in the hospices of course but also in the hospitals, insane asylums, and beggars' jails.[43] What La Rochefoucauld–Liancourt observed at Bicêtre in 1790 would long remain true for many other locations: "This building is at one and the same time a hospice, Hôtel-Dieu, boarding house, hospital, home for delinquents, prison, and correctional institution" (Report to the Committee on Beggary). As a consequence, the asylum system as envisaged by Pinel[44] would also affect the disabled, even if to a lesser degree than the insane: the medico-disciplinary order. It should be added that this order, too, was intended to provide rehabilitation. In these spaces assigned to aberrancy, "the double game of the totalitarian institution, to neutralize and rehabilitate at the same time, finds its best justification . . . exclusion and regimented life, these two strategies, are not mutually exclusive . . . the application, in a closed space, of a program of resocialization." Here rehabilitation and assistance are conjoined in the hard and circumscribed form that is the hospice-hospital, the official institution that will be dominated by medico-legal power of a moral and social kind, while awaiting the real specialization of later medicalization. The physician and the social reformer will enter into collusion, for they have agreed on a common "general social etiology" (Castel, *Les Métamorphoses de la question sociale,* 148), and they will progressively direct the policy of rehabilitation and assistance through *work,* always behind walls.

It is hard to resist quoting the last page of a chapter by Castel. He begins by himself citing the philanthropist Gerando. "It is not just a question, as one might otherwise think, of finding work for the poor; it is often a matter of educating them for work at all ages, that is, inspiring the taste for work, aiding them in developing the capacity for it, and forming the habit. It is not just a matter, as one might think, of achieving an economic goal . . . it is primarily a matter of achieving a moral goal . . . There is little speculative profit to be had from the products of such industry, but there is a great deal to be expected of its effects on the habits of the indigent, even when such speculation may be fruitless." Castel then continues: "Replace the word 'poor' by one of the multiple qualifications applied today to the various kinds of persons 'excluded' from the systems of exploitation and normalization and you will have the general formula for an assistance policy in a class society, with a place reserved for the various social and mental medicines, past, present, and to come. And also the key to the relationship of classical psychiatry to the problematics of labor. Not at all the recovery of an increase in value (except as a bonus), but rather the restoration of an order in which the extraction of surplus value may be the economic law, because subjection to the disciplines is its moral law."[45]

It is from within this medical *and* social logic, as typified in the psychiatry of alienation, that the celebrated law of June 30, 1838, pertaining to the insane was born. It regulated this domain for more than a century (until the birth of the sector system in the 1960s).[46] Castel, to quote him one more time, makes a very original analysis of this law that, at the very moment when it hands victory to the asylum as the unique solution, sounds the knell of alienation psychiatry in favor of a more modern discipline.

None of this will occur on behalf of the physically disabled. It is true that remediation and aid were applied in part in a social space of the asylum type and, in much milder fashion, in specialized institutions. The specialized institution is also a form of circumscription and of rigorous control of the aberrant. The specialized facility for the disabled shows the predominance of a social framework over a medical framework, although the one shapes the condition of the disabled no less than the other. This is why the conceptions of recovery and assistance are more adequate than those of exclusion and surveillance, which are the preferred approach to the mentally ill.

Testifying to this are the numerous services, especially those of a private nature, where the asylum system did not necessarily serve as model but where assistance and rehabilitation are in the fore. These establishments belong to the medical, and particularly the orthopedic, order. A frenzy for therapy seized numerous physicians and new techniques appeared and made rapid advances. We find, for example, orthopedic institutions such as that directed by Vincent Duval on rue Basse-Saint-Pierre in the Chaillot quarter of Paris,[47] which treated deformities of stature, club-feet, false ankylosis (stiffness) of the knee, chronic stiff necks, diseases of the joints. The disabled are residents there and the children receive

> all the prescribed lessons either from persons attached to the establishment or from outside teachers . . . Thus, this establishment is highly specialized, differing from those which admit every kind of illness, without concern for the antipathetic aspect of their grouping in a single location. There are even homes where they have also undertaken treatments of spinal misalignment, but the directors of these residences, lay or religious and foreign to the art of healing, are obliged to have recourse to outside physicians . . . Let us add that to mix young impaired subjects with others who have regular bodily properties is to expose them to humiliations that quickly lead to disappointment and distaste. (From Duval's prospectus)

The gap between this and the hospital formula is considerable. In addition, in these private institutions there prevailed an atmosphere, and standards of hygiene and shelter far superior to those of the hospital or hospice. "The costs of room and board, of necessity variable in accordance with the kind of treatment, its duration, etc., are determined by mutual agreement and according to a moderate fee schedule." This inclines one to think that only the well-to-do strata of society had access to the establishment.[48]

Thus a number of establishments with orthopedic objectives appeared; others worked with the idea of climate therapy, such as the first centers at Berck-sur-Mer or Forges-les-Bains for the "scrofulous."[49]

At these facilities, and at the hospitals too, important techniques were developed for straightening the body: the extension bed, which was to give rise to long discussions,[50] the use of electricity,[51] the appearance of the neck brace (Levacher), Scarpa's apparatus for clubfeet, a new conception of the corset,[52] the orthopedic swing—in short, a whole collection of *normalization devices* that are also signs of a new conception of motor skills and corporeality.[53]

The nineteenth century was a great era for orthopedics. Straightening out physically and straightening up behaviorally are put in the same semantic field, a normative one. Educate and rehabilitate, mind and body: draw upward, toward correctness. *Correct* is another keyword that forges a link between medicine and pedagogy. We witness the subtle shift from orthopedics to prosthetics.

For comparison with this French review, the wider European picture is furnished in the report of a commission established in 1896 by Louis Barthou, then minister of the interior.[54] The author first came into contact with institutions for the deaf or blind quite similar to those that sprang from the abbé de l'Épée or from Valentin Haüy. But it was in Sweden that he found it "apposite to cite societies for the assistance of the maimed and injured . . . To describe the organization of one of them is to introduce them all." The one he chose was called The Society for Assistance to the Maimed, Crippled, and Injured and was located in Göteborg. Its founder, the minister Hans Knudsen, said: "Idleness gives rise to the demoralization of the body and soul." From this we can imagine the program that was foreseen. Knudsen conceived of two establishments: an orthopedic polyclinic and, as a continuation, a vocational school. It is worth quoting an extended passage on the subject of this training school, since what is described there is so close to what was thought invented in France a half-century later.

As one might well expect, instruction at the Trade School is very different from that of schools attended by the able-bodied. The rules of conventional pedagogy are no longer applicable in an environment where the personnel is so dissimilar from the remainder of mankind. The whole art of the instructor who teaches a crippled person a craft or trade consists in developing in the latter the function of those limbs that are intact, bearing in mind the particular aptitudes of the individual. The nature, degree, and date of onset of the disability are also considerations in determining the best means of learning a trade. The great master here is experience.

Nor can ordinary tools be used in the majority of cases. Appropriate tools have had to be designed for various disabilities and to compensate for the part of the body that has been lost.

If we distinguish between bodily deficiencies and illnesses that reduce individual capacity, the maimed, crippled, and injured can be classed in four categories:

Those with a congenital deformity, for example, the one-armed;

The paralytics, as a consequence of diphtheria, scarlet fever, head injury, or a sickness affecting the spinal cord;

The accidentally maimed;

Individuals with generalized muscular weakness, caused by illnesses of the skeletal system and others.

To provide all these unfortunates with a trade, in the shortest time possible, is the objective of the teaching staff of the establishment. The staff is composed of female teachers for the supervision of general work and master tradesmen for the specialized apprenticeships. The trades that are most taught are, for men, cabinet-making, wood-working, wood sculpture, brush-making, chair-caning, shoe-making; for women, hand and machine sewing, knitting, crocheting, weaving.

The one-armed work with tools expressly designed for them, and sometimes they have recourse to an artificial hand or arm.

The student-worker is paid wages for his work, after covering the costs of his material.[55]

It is difficult to imagine the skill acquired by some of these disabled persons who have only a single useful hand but who have the use of their legs. There are some among them who, at the machine or lathe, work as quickly as the able-bodied and earn an equal wage.

When one of the students shows an aptitude for a trade that is not taught at the vocational school (clock-making, for example), the Society does not hesitate to make an extra outlay and pays the costs of a master craftsman in this line of work.

These students, with some few exceptions, are then placed with industries through the efforts of the Society. The Society even lends them the tools necessary for the exercise of their trade, on the condition that they be returned on the death of the beneficiary of the loan.

Neither willing nor able to assume a heavy financial burden, the Society gave up the idea of a residential school which would have been far too costly.

It does, however, come to the aid of the disabled who are taking courses and whose indigent state is known, by providing meals. The goods produced by the school are sold both at the school and during an annual exhibition held at Christmas. . . .

The report of the Gothenberg Society informs us that since October 3, 1885, the date of the opening of the school, until the month of May, 1897, the number of crippled trainees was 125, among whom 22 one-armed students (five were born without a forearm), and 17 paralytics incapable of using either arm. The other cripples were afflicted with more or less serious deformities which rendered difficult if not impossible their entry into an ordinary shop as apprentices.

Instruction in these schools for the crippled lasts from nine to ten months of the year.

Societies similar to that in Göteborg have been founded everywhere in Scandinavia: in Karlskrona in 1885, in Helsingborg in 1887, in Helsinki, Finland, in 1890, in Stockholm in 1891, in Christiania [now Oslo] in 1893.

The last-named, *Arbeidskole for Vanfore* (Vocational School for the Crippled) was set up a little too hastily in a building in Munkedams Veien, where hygiene was not held in very high esteem.

Nothing further need be added about the establishment in Stockholm after the outline that we have given of the organization and functioning of the Göteborg Society, nothing unless it be that it does not receive any subvention from the state nor from the municipality. This fact is not without importance.[56]

This picture from Sweden is quite exceptional and scarcely has parallels except for France, in the institutions for those with sensory impairments, and for England, where there were two foundations for disabled children.[57] This points emphatically to the new divide that will occur in the first decades of this century. But before these decades, the end of the nineteenth century marks a recovery of public assistance in France. In 1886 the Department of Assistance and Hygiene was created, in 1887 the Corps of Inspectors General, in 1888 the High Council for Public Assistance, all this crowned in 1889 by the International Council on Assistance, which would reaffirm the responsibility to provide help. Starting in these years, different initiatives (including a system of pensions) would be taken and would find their fulfillment in the law of July 14, 1905. In its first article, this law stipulates who shall receive assistance: "Every French citizen deprived of resources, incapable of providing through his work for the necessities of life and either older than 70 years of age or afflicted with a disability or a disease recognized as incurable." In its second article, the text states who is obliged to provide assistance: "Assistance is furnished by the municipality where the person aided has his subsidized residence; in the absence of a municipal home, by the department where the person aided has his departmentally subsidized residence; in the absence of any subsidized residence, by the state."

The third article, and here we have the essential of this law, responds to the question of the forms in which assistance is granted: "The aged, disabled, and incurable having a municipally or departmentally subsidized residence receive assistance at home. Those who cannot be usefully assisted at home are placed, if they consent, either in a public hospice, or in a private establishment, or with private persons, or finally in public or private establishments where lodging only, and independently of any other form of assistance, is assured them."

This law returns to the ideas of the Constituent Assembly, after the long wait of disability in a juridical no-man's-land. But it also shows the limits within which this century of explosive revolutionary liberties would keep itself and shows the effects of the terrible industrial yoke. A century that wished to educate (and compulsory schooling will be one of its fruits), that wished to restore (by moralizing and by technology)—a century that assisted, but initially through hospitalization and/or by protective and restrictive institutions.[58]

The centuries of French classicism were finally able to devise a solution to a problem that the Middle Ages had left wholly unresolved. The poor social integration (and the even less good spiritual integration at the close of the Middle Ages) became a relative civic integration underlying social marginalization.

To return to my habit of a final diagram, with all its impoverishment but also suggestiveness, I would say that the Middle Ages developed, particularly on the biological level, a notion of alterity with reference to the habitual and disengaged, in the narrow sense of the word, the concept of marginality, while on the ethical and social level all its attention was directed toward the fortune and misfortune of the disabled, seeking but never very successfully realizing a kind of sociability with them.

The classical centuries retain the biological perspective but introduce ideas of health and debility and thus acquire principles of classification. Ethics is less a factor, ceding to a vision that is initially social. The conforming and the aberrant—with reference to society—call for an act of separation, which corresponds to the ambition to classify. Let us summarize (and simplify) as follows:

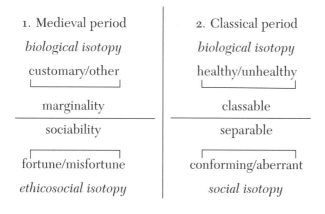

1. Medieval period	2. Classical period
biological isotopy	*biological isotopy*
customary/other	healthy/unhealthy
marginality	classable
sociability	separable
fortune/misfortune	conforming/aberrant
ethicosocial isotopy	*social isotopy*

6

The Birth of Rehabilitation

Effacement

The term *birth* cannot be used simply to pinpoint a new departure. It would be quite insufficient here to give an account of a beginning. A new way, both cultural and social, of addressing disability begins at the time of World War I. All the principal issues of our contemporary age, for this subject and others, are to be understood on the basis of this inception. The origins are interesting because of the consequences they will have. There is no value in simply reporting the event of a birth, but it is of compelling interest to analyze just what was initiated. In this sense, birth does not end until there is a new decisive rupture in the society in question or until a new society emerges. What are we dealing with when we speak of disability in the twentieth century and when we concern ourselves with it? How do we concern ourselves with it, how do we speak of it, and, from that, what new relationships are established between the disabled of earlier periods and present society? Discourse, image, praxis—and some in the medium of the others—what kind of light do they throw on the age-old problem of aberrancy? These questions are scarcely formulated before they risk getting away from us: are disability and handicap one and the same thing? What do we mean by society? Need we speak of aberrancy?

This new awareness of disability, this new revelation of the social fact, will be represented by the notion of *réadaptation*, "rehabilitation." Is the word sufficiently explicit to deal with the issues of the birth of which I speak? It has been trivialized, referring today to the collection of medical, therapeutic, social, and professional actions directed at those who are grouped under the generic term of disabled.

Phrases such as *la réadaptation des handicapés* "the rehabilitation of the disabled" become focal points, become slogans, typifying exactly the most established patterns of behavior. Other terms are also current, all iterative in nature (French equivalents of *retraining, readjustment*) but do not have the generality and pregnant quality of *réadaptation* in public discourse in France. This concept will be our point of reference.

This iterative term to designate the rehabilitation initiative, especially from the 1920s onward, is remarkable in its own right. It is applied to congenital cases as well as to the adventitious. It implies returning to a point, to a *prior* situation, the situation that existed for the able but one only postulated for the others. In any case, reference is to a norm. I shall later show how the a whole misleading vocabulary (*in-firme, in-valide, im-potent, in-capable,* etc.) was abandoned in favor of terms such as *handicapé.*

At the very moment that this dysphoric mode of designation was in the process of being deleted, the discourse of *retour,* "return," begins to appear. The lack is removed (words with negative prefixes in *in/m-* are erased) and reference is back to the assumed prior, normal state. This, then, is the act that shatters the received consensus, that puts an end to the preceding discourse, that generates the new specificity.

What happened that made this rupture possible? Who imposed a new regularity on the disability of the past? Of what series of actions is this practice of rehabilitation composed?

The first of these inquiries bears on which factors, socially, led the impaired to be considered as susceptible to rehabilitation. How did it happen that such discourse was made possible? The second inquiry has to do with schemes of thought that are specific to the era in which we live. In more semiotic language: we are seeking out the isotopies, the levels of reading that differ and cross one another in the typology under study. Finally, a third constituent is made up of the programs that are put in place for the disabled: what paths will they follow?

Without getting lost in terms of method, here then are three starting points from which we can address a number of problems, such as the following: Who are the agents who deal with disability and how do they proceed? How are fears, refusals, and acceptances formulated today? What kind of discourse is generated on the causes, categories, and degrees of disability? In short, to take into account the major inquiry, which is at the same time the day-to-day question, what do we do, *really*, and "really" means symbolically as well, with the disabled in Western society?

The Moment—The Conditions

At the close of what the European nations called the Great War without knowing to what extent this qualifier was relative, a startling number of men were discharged injured for life. They were called *mutilés de guerre* "maimed war veterans" on the model of those disabled by accidents at work.[1] The "mutilated" were not only amputees. Mutilation applied to all alteration of integrity, of integralness. It amounted to a degradation, but one by removal—or deterioration—which has the effect of suppression. The maimed person is someone missing something precise, an organ or function. Thus, the first image presented by this change in terminology is that of damage. The war has taken away, we must replace. The development of the "pro-sthesis" dates from this war.

A National Office of the War Maimed (*Office national des mutilés*) was created on March 2, 1916, and is today the National Veterans Office (*Office national des anciens combattants*). It would initiate the general use of prostheses and would, moreover, exercise absolute control in this domain through the supply of this equipment, and through control of the approval for reimbursement of costs. Until just before the war of 1914–18, only the crutch and wooden leg were employed as prostheses, even if some ingenious inventors had anticipated artificial hands, for example.[2]

But prosthesis is not only the pieces of wood, iron, now plastic that replace the missing hand or foot. It is also the very idea that you can *replace.* The image of the maimed person and of the society around him becomes prosthetic. Replacement, re-establishment of the prior situation, substitution, compensation—all this now becomes possible language.

To this first feature, generated by the war, is to be added what people said and felt about the war itself with respect to the wounded. It was nothing less than a catastrophe: a terrible, abrupt event, as dictionaries define it. But catastrophe does not generate aberrancy. Catastrophe can be the object of repair; we rebuild after an earthquake. To these "soldiers, husbands, and fathers of families" who left part of themselves behind in combat, the others owe a debt.[3] Culpability and moral obligation are linked with the idea of catastrophe; we can and must repair, re-establish, restore, in other words, efface, expiate, redeem. The wound can be closed in a scar. The war, like employment itself, can destroy and diminish, but restoration, incorporation, insertion are necessary and possible. A new will is born: to reintegrate.[4] Everyone knows that the basic ideas here are of the integral, intact, complete, at the same time as recovering possession of a former place, a prior situation, property of the past. When speaking of the war-wounded, we are also speaking of rehabilitation. And, inversely, speaking of rehabilitation envisages disability as a lack to be filled, almost a lack to be overcome.

But, you will say, we are only talking of the victims of war (another designation for the maimed, which refers to another level of language, this time moral and religious). It is here that we can see the break between the two eras: the war-injured will take the place of the disabled; the image of disability will become one of an insufficiency to be made good, a deficiency to eradicate. This is a new notion, as the appearance of legislative discourse and a multitude of institutions testify. This is a notion different from cure. Cure is a removal and relates to health. Rehabilitation is situated in the social sphere and constitutes replacement for a deficit. Giving voice to this shift will be one of the functions of the new language of disability. Lastly, rehabilitation becomes a generalized notion and will be extended to all the disabled, to all forms of disability. In the 1920s a swing will occur and a new logic will come to predominate.

Legislative Discourse or Assimilation

The 1914 war provides a reference point, nothing more, but nothing less. That is to say, it was not the only determinant but it marked the turning point at the significant moment in a new mental and social division.

But this event was preceded by others just as important: accidents at work toward the close of the nineteenth century. This issue was given a juridical solution by the passage of the law of April 9, 1898, on victims of work-related accidents. It was extended on October 27, 1919, to illnesses of vocational origin, then to the agricultural sector on December 16, 1922, and to people working in the home, August 2, 1923.

Today, I would attach more importance to policies that originated with those who suffered accidents at work than to those for the war-wounded. Even if it is true on the one hand that it was the question of wounded veterans that established the concept of rehabilitation and put in place vocational redeployment, and thus reintegration (not least economic) into society, on the other hand the ideas of compensation, collective responsibility, state involvement, normalization based on a perception of the average, and social insurance had their origins in work-related accidents.[5]

Juridical discourse on these matters first appeared in the last decades of the nineteenth and first decades of the twentieth century.[6] This incipient legislation was doubtless linked to middle-class practices of *good works* (often by women), and was paternalistic, Catholic, burdened with culpability but also reform-minded, at times lucid, often good-hearted. Heading this list of characteristics is the concept of *assistance*. The connection, however, is not at all simple. If one is to believe certain critics, assistance is more significantly related to social control of populations. Assistance, in this sense, would far outlast the distinctive features of the French bourgeoisie of the nineteenth century.

I shall state here what I accept and what I must reject of the extremely well executed and very lucid work of Jeannine Verdes-Leroux, since I shall employ her terminology. Her study is more detailed than mine, since she subdivides the twentieth century into a number of segments: charitable assistance for the education of the uncultivated, creation of a social monitoring system with notions of re-integration, rationalism, and specialization in order to contain the excluded. But her book has a single thesis, which leaves less room for analysis than my study, where divisions are on a larger scale. Her thesis is that social work, under more and more elaborate and concealed forms, is progressively coming into the hands of the dominant class and is each day increasingly the intermediary for a division of social classes, to the detriment of the urban working class. It is just this systematization that will not be followed in the following pages. There is the sense of stereotype in the thesis, as in the discourse of political parties. Verdes-Leroux sees a multitude of details with great clarity, especially the direction that social services have recently taken: psychological treatment of cases, which obliterates the material conditions; recognition of "maladapted" social strata in order to anticipate their reactions; the provision of employment to a multitude of agents of the middle class; exploitation of the theme of the excluded in order to nourish an ideology of social defense[7]—in short, a fluid and generalized vision of maladjustment and a return to positions like those of Pinel, which justify more than ever the kinds of actions undertaken. Verdes-Leroux's study encompasses the whole of social work. Considering only the question of the disabled, my comments are obviously less general but may well be more incisive.

It is common sense to state that an attitude—or a discourse or an institution—can survive, occasionally long survive, the conditions that gave rise to it. Inversely, certain intuitions, certain premonitions may come well before the establishment of a practice. It is thus, in our case, that the idea of responsibility and compensation appears in legislation dominated by the concept of assistance. Business is liable for the accident caused by and at work and it is obligated to compensate the injury.[8] At a time when assistance pure and simple was at its zenith, obligations more properly *social* than moral began to insinuate themselves. But it is necessary to add at once that if assistance passed to the second rank and left the first rank to integration,[9] but without ever disappearing and leading to all kinds of future contradictions, the ideas of responsibility and of compensation did not prove dominant either.

This shows that rehabilitation is no longer assistance, but for all that has not become more just.

Rehabilitation shoots up as a new phenomenon, overshadowing the modest growth of social equity, and brings to an end a first period of aid. What constituted rehabilitation at this time?

The first period of assistance that I am speaking of can be associated with class struggle. In fact, in the heyday of liberalism this association was quite overt. The poor were to be raised up—above all, morally. With this act of recovery, an effort was made to impose on everyone the models of the middle class, its style of life, and its conduct. But the cultural scheme of assistance is not tied to the appearance of the "classist" phenomenon of the nineteenth century. Its roots lie deeper, in the sense of a destiny and in an almost ontological vision of society: the poor constitute an ongoing, inevitable category, intrinsic to all societies. Since the Middle Ages, the idea of assistance has been present because there was no analysis of poverty as socially produced, a production that is still ongoing. Middle-class liberalism of the last century was also heir to this frozen, fixated conception. But liberal assistance, in contrast to strictly charitable assistance, consists of having the poor adopt liberalism's values.

Rehabilitation is in opposition to assistance on two earlier identified fronts: the poor are to be *reintegrated* and it is less a question of assimilation to middle-class models than coercive association with certain styles of life, even though domination continues in this other way as well. On the cultural level, it appears ineffective to commiserate and patronize; henceforth it is better to "do as if" (as if . . . there were no longer any difference). In any case, even though this opposition did not characterize all the sectors covered by social action, it did show itself to be relevant in the area of disability. The juridical discourse that flourished from the years of the First World War reveals this amply and proves the point.[10] All the *civil disabled,* with the tubercular patients at their head, are now progressively and continuously more closely identified with the war-wounded. Tuberculosis remained the great fear until the 1950s. Then the developmentally impaired were so identified, and finally the social cases.

The field of mutilation extends indefinitely, thus also that of malad-justment, then reintegration, finally rehabilitation. If we question what differentiates the concepts of "re-" that have rather haphazardly been used up to this point, I would say that they come at logical intervals: to reintegrate, we must redeploy; to redeploy, we must retrain; to retrain, we must rehabilitate (the body and its organs, intellect and movement). But there is another way of sequencing all this: we can replace what is missing, and this leads to retraining, and that to redeploying then to reintegrating, and that is rehabilitation. Along this axis of specific actions, rehabilitation always comes at the end, as the most specific action or as the most generic. Rehabilitation is co-extensive with disabilities and their extension in time. Little by little, starting with the post-war years, a conceptual fuzziness takes over, one that will end up in the word *handicap,* and a single intention will come to dominate: every impaired person becomes, like the war-wounded, someone who lacks a place and not just an organ or a faculty, someone for whom a place has to be made. Not a place offering sociability or a place in social networks but simply in society, in the social fact. Indeed, other, earlier eras and societies never failed to *situate* the disabled and their disabilities, but few if any ever had the ambition, pretension, and intention to relocate them in the machinery of production, consumption, work, and play in the day-to-day community. For good or ill, the disabled were exceptions and stood for exceptionality, alterity; now that they have become ordinary, they have to be returned to ordinary life, to ordinary work. They no longer represent anything that is *other;* they simply serve to identify a socioeconomic technique that is still not sufficiently developed, but which hopes to solve the problem. They have simply become "different," but this complicates the problem in a rather different way.[11] This takes us infinitely farther than a question of social class: rehabilitation marks the appearance of a culture that attempts to complete the act of identification, of making identical. This act will cause the disabled to disappear and with them all that is lacking, in order to assimilate them, drown them, dissolve them in the greater and single social whole. This desire for fusion, for confusion, is more serious, more submerged than an ideological strategy; it is an index, and an important one, of a slow slide toward a society that is less and less pluralist, more and more rigid.

To content oneself with denouncing this fact by referring it to the problem of the relationship between dominant and dominated classes is not only a simplification, but it also serves to reinforce the phenomenon in question. In fact, people exclaim about those who, like myself, do not seek to reduce this reintegration to a well-known process in Marxist theory. Here I am on the side of the dominant trying to conceal the domination, since I am saying that the negation of difference is a cultural fact that is shared by all classes and since I am saying that it is perhaps a serious matter to wish to efface differences. To be orthodox, I would have to say: the dominant want to erase differences through assimilation to themselves, while equality and access on the part of everyone to the same goods, values, and liberties are what is required. What I have against this language, which is more militant than analytical, is that it does not go far enough in its criticism. Certainly, the reintegration process is also implicated in the class struggle, but it goes infinitely farther. It is society as a whole that no longer wants to see the facts, and it is a very different matter than a refusal of equality.

I admit that things are clearer for disability than for other defects; the first directive, in many respects, was to control and monitor. Rehabilitation certainly participates in the powerful action of maintenance that is social action, but here, however, the primary concern was to efface.

In saying this, I can sense the thousands of objections that will be raised. I shall take up two of them: effacement hardly describes the social will that specialized internment, labels, rejections offer us . . . in short, specifics that were never achieved. The effacement is of such little significance that we can carefully distinguish the categories of those who can be reintegrated from those that we are simply content to support (or, more recently, to aid, which is a very different thing), a policy which is widespread and tolerated even more than in the preceding decades. These two claims cannot be challenged or dismissed except by the analyses of the institutions and their language that now follow. Before turning my gaze from legislation, a little comic relief can be had by examining its most recent product, the law of 1975.[12] Seen from the point of view of content, the discourse is meager: it rearranges by complexifying. It is discourse that inaugurates nothing, creates nothing, neither concepts, nor institutions, nor processes. The little specialists who prowl around their offices in the ministries can take a few trifles for a new heaven and earth, even though there is nothing to them. But seen from the angle of its connection with other legislative discourse, it takes on distinctive signification.[13] In the sphere of mental illness the knell has sounded for internment, although confinement has not disappeared. Guardianship can be substituted for internment. This procedure, milder than that of "voluntary commitment" (i.e., by a third party!) and based on the evaluation, without definite criteria, of a judge predisposed to the institution of guardianship, puts mental illness back in the immense field of other incapacities. Intellectual diminution no longer needs to be enclosed; it can live and be returned to the everyday run of things. But the deficiency is not allowed to go unchecked: physicians, judges, social workers provide control, proper functioning. Remunerative work is thus given to a greater number of agents. But the discovery lies in this: the measure of irrationality in the asylum system appears substantial faced with the fine pragmatic system of the social labor market.[14] The alterity of unreason—that reason had revealed and defined and taken precautions against (and enjoyment from!)[15] by means of confinement—can be controlled without systematic sequestration. Neither shameful nor even abnormal, it is a commodity: administrative and commercial reasoning tames it better than the reflective reason of another age. The Age of Reason, the Enlightenment, just as well called the Age of Madness,[16] was very metaphysical; it produced confinement, then the asylum.[17] Our age is technocratic and mercantile: it will soon have no need of physical exclusion.

The juridical discourse of 1975 employed the term *handicapé* to cover all maladjustments linked to deficiencies, the latter unspecified. Power was concentrated in groupings of specialists and social workers who were the deciding instances in terms of the placement (i.e., place to be assigned) of each individual concerned. These ruling commissions have a tendency to prefer, for the most part, direct solutions of redeployment, without appealing to specialized places and processes. It is possible to entirely avoid anything that resembles exclusion. And financial reasons can be cited at the same time.[18] But this is neo-

assistance, very far, it is true, from that of the past, and consists of a general assumption of responsibility and authority on the social level, with all categories mixed together. That is, limitations are very carefully put on formulas for training of any duration in order, on completion, to place trainees in appropriate jobs, in sheltered establishments, or even with the specialized agents of regulatory institutions. The commissions to which reference is here made are of two kinds, although all are run by regional governments: commissions for the special education of children and adolescents (Commissions d'éducation spéciale [CDES]) and technical commissions for the counseling and vocational redeployment of adults (Commissions techniques d'orientation et de reclassement professionnel [Cotorep]). Every disabled person who wishes to be so recognized, in order to benefit from specialized structures and processes, must come before one or another of these agencies. Their administrative complexity is very great. Only the smallest part of their counseling concerns vocational training; after that come sheltered workshops and finally what is called direct placement. "Sheltered workshop" is a formula for the employment of the disabled and is assisted according to two very distinct models.

In order to decipher the primary (and hidden) role of the agencies of which I am speaking, I see them intended to fulfil the function of the cosmetic surgeon: looking after the social face. Losing face is the worst thing that can happen to a society that has stopped being metaphysical, that has stopped seeing itself as powerless before certain misfortunes, which has succeeded in making alterity disappear. The face must be smoothed over: it is more than ever the age of appearances. Behind this made-up face, the disparities, contradictions, and roughness remain, and people know it. To treat these difficulties, we have good, proven prescriptions, such as classic psychiatry and vocational rehabilitation which go hand in hand with repressive or segregationist forms. But these treatments are no longer supposed to be seen: the disabled person can be among us and pass unnoticed. But she is carefully, although more invisibly, taken in hand, and thus monitored and directed. There is a strong logical connection between the first juridical steps of the 1920s and the most recent law. Giving substance to the concept of rehabilitation (= the demand to be like the others), this legislation has now completed the movement toward indistinctness and dilution. But this is also a beginning: will those persons who demand rehabilitation be prepared to accept the final consequences? Exactly what in fact will erasure and deletion require to be fully realized?

Clearly, we must concede that the movement of social forgetfulness is still in its early, unformed stages. I admit as well that much as I believe that my analysis of the present cultural trend is soundly based, I see resistance in daily praxis to this trend. But in my eyes it is undeniable that the demand to be "like the others" has been, in the most deceptive of ways, so managed by legislation and the institutions that the cry will soon be heard, "We're disabled too!" The trick consists in this: in a liberal, prosperous, and technologically advanced society, means can be found so that the disabled no longer appear different. They will be admitted on the condition that they are perfectly assimilated to the able-bodied. This assimilation may initially take the form of a sustained exclusion: limited resources, specialized institutions, separate work places, etc. But the moment will come when exclusion is no longer a problem: it is itself working on behalf of effacement. The time will come when the disabled will no longer be able to raise their voices and many will no longer have the desire or the taste to do so. What are you complaining about? What would we complain about? Complaint becomes impossible, this is the direction in which we are going. "If you are like everybody else, even though you got here by a detour, why should you have anything to say?"

I am not saying that exclusion will disappear. I am saying that the problem of our society is not a failure to integrate but of integrating too well, integrating in such a way that identicalness reigns, at least a rough identity, a socially constructed identity, an identity of which citizens can be convinced. That is to say, when we know the strength of a consensus, there is an identity no less real than if it had actually been achieved, for social imaginings are just as effectively social as the material or objective situation of things and people.

We have to localize the benefits over the longer course of contemporary Western society. Legal and institutional arrangements have improved the lot—and thus also relieved the subjectivity—of people we call disabled. It would be absurd to entertain a nostalgia for some fancied Middle Ages. It is not a question here of moral judgment or simply an estimation of the relative happiness of people. This is not what it's about. The question is to know what cultural cost we will have to pay for our advanced technology, and above all it is a question of remaining lucid about the direction in which we are steered by any policy that is put in place. Is the integration that has been carried out successful? What kind of integration are we talking about? The integration foreseen by laws, administrations, and institutions seems to me an integration of oblivion, of disappearance, of conformity, of normalization. Under what conditions has this become imaginable, possible? Through these demands, still infrequent and dispersed, I can see appearing rehabilitation policies and temporal horizons that differ from the proposed integration. But before considering this future scenario, let's continue our analysis of the present situation. It is important to underline the simple fact of a piece of legislation, just as important as its legal contents. It is quite evident that to legislate is the equivalent, in almost every domain, to making things more complicated and to centrism, the centralization of political power. This trend is increasingly pronounced in our time. This also corresponds to the technological and directive character of industrial society. To legislate is to impose a norm, a code of the universalist type on phenomena and practices which until then had been left on their own, to their diversity, empiricism, even their anarchy. A common order is thenceforth imposed. As a consequence, disability is elevated to an existence and a consistency that it never had. Now disability is raised to prominence, when it was earlier seen as assimilated, as self-evident, or as a minor matter. The "thing" has been designated, defined, framed. Now it has to be scrutinized, pinpointed, dealt with. Criteria, stages, regulations are attached. People with "it" make up a marked group, a social entity. Now, those who were formerly disparate and objects of the acts of the kind-hearted do have rights but they are named with a specificity that constitutes an identifying marker. Moreover, if we examine the rights that have been accorded them, they are only those that all citizens have and that have never been the object of any formal declaration: the right to work, the right to education, the right to a guaranteed economic life, and so on. For the disabled, these rights are *stated,* promulgated. Left out of the common lot, it must be affirmed that they are still part of it. This is giving them a status, but is just as much, to play with words a bit, to set them up like statues. The disabled, henceforth of all kinds, are *established as a category to be reintegrated and thus to be rehabilitated.* Paradoxically, they are designated in order to be made disappear, they are spoken in order to be silenced. This is a contradiction, of course, but has its basis in the play between being and seeming in our society. The more their social elimination becomes possible, the more their medical, psychological, even sociological existence is affirmed. This is how the mirage is produced: the publicly stated numbers and mass are in proportion to the credibility being sought for the claim that the problem is really being solved. What is more, undifferentiated pleading for the excluded and affirming "their rights to share in national solidarity" by means of a law—as a consequence putting them in quotation marks—is to expand social work and appeal to the bottomless goodwill of governments and citizens.[19] The moment when being and appearing are publicly manifest is followed by that in which there is no appearing. We have often enough heard, "Today, so much has been done for the disabled," and we see that these statements are disseminated at every opportunity.[20] All the arrangements that have been made do not in the least signify that they are assumed to be adequate. Concern for them, preoccupation with them has never been so intense: their existence, in this sense, is not in question and is generally recognized. But the preoccupation has to do with social leveling, not initially with domination and control, but rather with an immersion. Society homogenizes, even when based on classes in struggle, even based on recognized particularities. This is perhaps the most subtle paradox that society has managed to sustain in these times. The culture of "as if," the civilization of the secret are making great strides.

Finally, in the juridical discourse initiated in the third decade of this century, we would do well to test out a huge unthought thought, which I call the principle of the empirical norm. In fact, the so-called disabled person, the invalid, is evaluated and evaluates himself with reference to others, the valid ones. Imitation of the able, equality with them (even competition), such is the tension that runs through rehabilitation, since the legislative texts raise the possibility of a residence of one's own, a job, social mobility, etc., "like everybody else." This is to say that the ghetto has been abolished, even if many accommodations, on a variety of registers, are still to come. But this affirms that everything has been polarized with relation to "like everyone else." The defective takes the ordinary as model, and success consists in being able to drive a car, live in a big apartment, work eight hours a day, go on summer holidays, and so on. Being ironical about the desire for autonomy is out of the question, whether it be the autonomy of daily acts and work, or financial autonomy. The numerous accounts—always highly affective communications—of those who have been able to give expression to the onerous victory that is the recovery or acquisition of these elementary acts cut short all criticism. What I am saying here is very different. Rehabilitation—without anyone paying attention to it or resisting it, rehabilitation as a fact—accepts as its norm the empirical norm. The very name alone indicates this. The most widely held belief is, in fact, that if you devote sufficient resources, it is possible to reduce the distance and bring each person, however great the burden she carries, to reoccupy a normal place in the group of the able (the normal). We then see appear on the level of technologies of substitution, apparatuses that permit, for example, the deaf and those with cerebral palsy, otherwise completely abandoned, to learn the means of communication, language, life relationships, even a vocation. On the administrative and legal level, we have seen appear arrangements to permit the access of the disabled to employment.[21] We have seen specialized services appear on the educational level, specialized formulas of all kinds to provide schooling, training, socialization. The pedagogical conceptions vary, the strategies are at times contradictory, the underlying ideologies draw their inspiration from different intellectual soil. But everyone agrees on this point: even when everything is set to brake the process, readjustment must be to society as society is presently constituted. Certainly, the actors on the scene bring thousands of charges against each other—and these charges are often very serious and very important. One of these is made between those who attribute to the powers that be—the powers at the interior of each particular organization as well as public authorities—an intention and passive stance (conscious or unconscious) that will leave the excluded to their exclusion, and these same powers who view their antagonists as inciters to revolution, irresponsible dreamers. In short, a political struggle develops, at times supported by political and labor organizations. But these struggles are all in tacit agreement on the concept of an empirical norm. In the Middle Ages, we have seen, the disabled were so "other" that, like all the poor, they were located in a state that was socially and quasi-ontologically different. There are, as there always will be, rich and poor, able and less able. In our times, it's a bit the other way around: in order to free the disabled from their unfortunate fate, they are considered subject to the same rights and possibilities as others. There are to be no more abnormal situations; it is no longer acceptable that psychological, mental, or physical differences create the breach that they did. The gap must be filled. There is no better way to escape the fear of strangeness than by forgetting aberrancy through its dissolution into the social norm. It is all a question of knowing whether this undertaking is really possible. Isn't this where the great innovation lies in comparison with the classical period as described by Foucault? Rehabilitation has moved out in front of the hospital (from which it derives, so this is only logical). In principle, it shuts the door on the practice of internment. But to open the door on what? On to the negation of disability through adjustment, integration. It entails fusing abnormality with the normality that is established and recognized by social consensus. We are obliged to note that this constitutes a new confinement. Specificity and aberrancy are thereby forbidden and condemned. The different must be folded into the commonplace, into the accepted, into the recognized. This is aimed at resolving two problems: fear and sequestration.

From the social perspective, this image of the disabled as beings to be rehabilitated signifies that society sees itself as a single order to be maintained; it sees itself as having the duty, the mission, the task of voiding disparities into its norm. A frequent reaction offers an example. For a long time, let's say the last fifty years, the right of the disabled to work has been proclaimed, and considerable efforts have been undertaken to achieve this end. But this has still not really happened. Today, when the value of work is questioned and many in the younger generation categorically distance themselves from the ideology of work—very interiorized among the working classes—certain disabled persons attempt to win support to have their new claims recognized: work is not the only form of rehabilitation. Why oblige people to expend so much effort, to accept so many constraints (in training, separation from families, specialized programs in residence, etc.) simply to be reduced to low-income salaried employees, scarcely receiving more than if they were on welfare, and contributing to a vast consumer-oriented production that is more and more insipid and alienating? In the face of such an attitude, what do the rehabilitation agencies have to say? They would certainly reply that it is imprudent to abandon the goal of employment, given our present social instability and the even more pronounced precariousness of disabled persons; that the risk of being forced to have recourse to welfare assistance pure and simple is too fraught with consequences. But, above everything else, there will surely be this answer: it is not up to disabled people to change society; if society were to change and become another—a society of leisure for example—then they could claim these same rights not to work, they could demand total choice. But disability cannot be a confrontational position, a force for social change, a mutant or revolutionary minority. In other words, the disabled should always adapt to society such as it is. The debate has started up again in this last decade of the twentieth century, in which the problem I have called exclusion (increases in unemployment, increasing disaffection) has repercussions for the problem of disability, not only to bring this sector into question but also to invite it to enter more fully into the larger social debate. To me it seems certain that disability, based on what has been called positive discrimination, shares the curious agenda of some officially recognized minority groups, no doubt for fear of losing a hard-won specificity or in any case of seeing it again become stakes in the game. This has been in order to avoid two extremes: a too-narrow claim for specificity, or dissolution into problems of a too-general nature.

Thus, figuring disability as an anomaly to be made to disappear through integration into social conformity is to represent society, empirically given, as a norm not to be transgressed, as a sort of universal capable of assuming, through annulment, all differences. In certain forms of society, like that of the Middle Ages, the difference that the disabled and simple interjected was so little manageable that it was given an atemporal quality, so that either society lived with it in a charitable relationship or organized it into a specific order of being (the leprosariums). But the social fabric supported and permitted this strangeness without being able to reduce it, without undertaking any action truly to integrate it, that is, through institutional means. In our society—entrepreneurial and technically efficient, essentially active, imperial—the difference is erased (I am speaking on the level of the present fresh will and not, for the moment, on that of the contradictions of this society), but society, in its leveling effects, is posited as a unidimensional order of ethicoeconomic character into which all must be resolved.

Institutional Discourse or Imitation

Legislation is conceivable only with the support of widespread uniform behavior and established praxis. Will the day-to-day activity of rehabilitation say the same thing as the juridical voice whose speaker can scarcely be made out? It is hardly easier, on this institutional ground, to make out *who* is speaking?

Before the war of 1914–18, and this will confirm this rupture as our reference point, there existed only the psychiatric institutions on one side and some establishments for those with sensory impairment on the other. The latter were not connected with the asylum. They sprang up beside it, even in opposition to it. For someone aware of the history of the treatment of insanity, this is not surprising at first glance: the "mad" were isolated, both on the level of the knowledge that was available (or that was projected) of mental disorder and on the level of institutions. By the end of the nineteenth century the asylum was firmly in place. Alienation was the ruling concept: medicalization would be added to this moral and social action; internment is henceforth the preferred and single form of intervention; the expert psychiatrist, absolute master of the rationalized space of the asylum where all madness ends up, the benevolent leader of the phalanxes of citizens without rights,[22] is one of the quintessentially important personages of society. The physically disabled are not in the asylum and the sequestration of the mentally ill puts an end to the mixture of the two categories. Establishments for the bodily deficient will not be born of the asylum system. Otherwise, rehabilitation will strive to free from the asylums, in particular from the "old people's homes," many impaired persons who had been taken for mentally ill because they showed identical symptoms.[23]

This separation, however, introduces a question: from an epistemological point of view, are retraining centers that different from asylums? The large establishment of Berck-Plage, for example, founded for the treatment of tuberculosis patients, did it not recreate the space of the asylum? All those designated and selected by medical expertise were collected as if in a zoo and left to wander in a universe of illness. There was neither school nor culture nor contact with the world of the healthy. But since the interned subjects were of a different kind than in the asylums, abrupt action was possible. In this sense rehabilitation was born in opposition to the asylum model. Are we justified, however, in historically separating rehabilitation from the treatment of madness? . . . and separating the physically disabled from the mentally deficient? Today, when the same legislation affects them all together, when institutions are so similar to one another, when the boundaries are often indistinct, how are we to speak of this century that is about to close, which from a divorce made a union?[24]

But the connections between mental affliction and physical illness are not everything. The former focused the attention of the classical age and the nineteenth century just as today it attracts almost exclusive concern. But the latter is doubtless no less relevant. The lame, amputees, the chronically ill, hunchbacked, deaf, blind, and others were offered services destined for the mass of the poor, among which the *hôpital général* and the hospices . . . unless their disability could be exploited in some practical or profitable way, or the circumstances of their birth permitted them to escape public charity. But all this stopped the day when the blind gained access to writing through Louis Braille. This was the passage to a fundamentally altered situation, in the wake of which Maurice de Sizeranne conceived of a great association for the blind and there was a flowering of organizations, albeit a half-century later. This put an end to the lack of differentiation— before it was rediscovered.

The disabled were no longer simply the poor. The disabled began to stand out against the mixed background of misery. They also stood in contrast to mental disorders of all kinds but only to see themselves stationed like these troubled persons, as a world apart, with a marked perimeter. The shortsightedness of the asylum system haunted subsequent initiatives without policymakers becoming conscious of it. Ambivalence lay in the juxtaposition of marginality and its suspension; it designates but conceals; when the ambivalence ends, the demonstrative element increases before the veil finally falls. The disabled had been lost in the mass of the indigent; now they are recognized, shown consideration, and put to one side in order to be made "like everyone else"! It was not inevitable that specialized institutions and establishments should emerge. Italy, for one, is an exception in this regard. Was it that the asylum model, as if stuck to the social unconsciousness, had become an obsession? Proximity and distance are the alternating stages in the evolution of the asylum and of the "center" for the disabled. As witness, beyond the historical origins just referred to, note the curious influence of the centers on the asylum. It would not be until the mid-1930s that an institution would be founded for the rehabilitation of the psychologically disabled on the model of those for physical deficiencies.[25] The rehabilitation of the mentally ill *followed* that of the disabled. Was it this, well after the first doubts about the law of 1838,[26] that shook the psychiatric edifice? However much this may have been the case, the abrupt break cannot be attributed to this form of rehabilitation,[27] but the gap it created had nothing to do with it. From another perspective, just as psychiatric institutions started to become more flexible, rehabilitation centers (for both the mentally and physically ill) found their position strengthened. Is this a new moment in this history of proximity and distance?

It is true that there exist two kinds of structures for mental disorders today (and here rehabilitation must be recognized as the parent): the psychiatric hospital, which took over from the asylum and still resembles it, and remedial centers for the developmentally retarded,[28] centers that are a good deal more ambivalent, since they have been sufficiently psychiatrized to remain the monopoly of doctors, but have a strong scholastic and vocational stamp. Half sequestration, half a conventional residential school, a good image of them can be had from the many documentary films. *A Child Is Waiting* is an exposé of the inevitable character of institutionalization, when no-one—neither family nor school nor the isolated individual—can live with mental illness. Of necessity, recourse must be had to the establishment directed by a hard-nosed humanist, an enlightened but principled teacher, devoted to his task, courageous in the face of a central administration that is ignorant and repressive—in short, the very type of those who direct rehabilitation. Men on the cusp of two worlds, two cultures: the universe of control over differences, politically engaged, scientifically based, and the universe of singularities, supported by real sociability and guided by knowledge without totalitarianism. The double structure, hospital/therapy center, only partly covers the conceptual distinction psychological/developmental. It is evident that foundations for the mentally ill were oriented toward mental deficiency and not toward insanity.[29] But the paths get confused quickly in this domain (what is autism?); the positions, intervention programs, and institutions overlap, send their clients back and forth. Today, rehabilitation in this domain is a good key for unlocking the universe of the asylum as it continues to implement measures initiated in the 1970s: greater dispersal but more discrete administration.

What was the discourse of the institutions intended for the disabled when they first arose? The same. The rampant growth and not just blooming of institutions—the chronology offers the proof[30]—is a consequence of the policies of 1945, in particular the celebrated founding legislation for social security. Although mismanaged in the following decades, its initial orientation was based in an effective and proportional solidarity among citizens and in a quite complete and thorough assumption of responsibility for care in order to prevent the development of inegalitarian insurance systems. The invention and widespread application of what was called "social coverage" provided the effective means and incarnated the desire for reintegration that was already present. For any contemporary history of social gains and of the labor movement in particular, 1945 is a threshold year and its consequences are the severe tension between a struggle to develop what had been won and political entropy. But from the cultural point of view that I have adopted, 1945 simply quickens the pace. Indeed, it should be noted, before returning to the real birth of rehabilitation, that the health dimension—which experienced a major and successful expansion in the form of hospitals— was outstripped tenfold by the extension of social security. This is why institutions for troubled youth and more generally for the mentally impaired experienced growth only after World War II. The means that were being offered? Old school psychiatry. And so psychiatrization had its heyday. And this is testimony to a contradiction to which I shall return: the will to rehabilitate would be held back by the power of exclusion and internment that was inherited from the past; its return was possible thanks to the resources for social protection, more exactly in health, that were available after 1945.

The positive or negative character of the way in which these notorious regulations were exploited is not my subject; in fact, instead of favoring the cumbersome hospital structure, a health program much closer to individuals could have been carried out with the same resources and could thus have demedicalized this program. What I reproach at the moment is that the post-war period only caused the bursting of a fruit that was already swollen and overripe, without ejecting the old worm of exclusion.

Let us return to the 1920s to examine the patterns of thought that informed the first large associations that sprang up. I shall select as my archetype—although she was not chronologically the first[31]—Suzanne Fouché, a young woman who uttered her cry from her gurney at Berck-Plage in 1929. Here she is, calling for the economic independence of the sick and, to accomplish this, the right to reintegration into the labor force, which presupposes vocational rehabilitation. There was an article, then a conference, then a foundation bearing her name that became a rallying cry.[32] Admittedly, only aid to the physically afflicted was foreseen at the time, but the idea would spread. The scheme is simple but eloquent: not to leave out of active and productive life those who have experienced misfortune, but to furnish them with the means to be once again citizens and workers "like the rest," or according to a later slogan "fully." This amounts to bearing one's disability as an individual trial, more or less spiritualized; this amounts to resigning oneself to it, in fact, to accepting society's margins. But at the same time, acquiescence to an indelible difference disappears.

Now the wish to be "like everyone else" takes over, a move is made to rejoin the group of the able . . . at the same time as the conditions of industrial society are raised so as to be compatible only with normal persons. Good or bad, with varying emphasis and means, all the initiatives, all the actions that came into being "on behalf of the disabled" are reduced to the example that we gave as the archetype: the fall into reintegration among the crowd of normals. It remains a large-scale action toward the *ultimate* effacement of the disabled, no matter how vigorous the intervening recognition of specificity. The practice of "rehabilitation" is constructed on this conception: the maladjustment at the starting point is to be compensated for so that the end point is adjustment. Starting with afflictions considered simply physical but then looking into mental, psychological, and social injuries and impairments, a multitude of associations, groups, actions, and publications have appeared in the last sixty years to cover the whole field of maladjustment. I would emphasize how much "non-thought" there is in the new attitude, in the form of the assumption of empirical normalcy. But I have already made this analysis concerning legislative discourse. I shall show the collusion, not by chance, between this recognition of a norm accepted as a given, and the liberalism of the social class that has economic and political power. But, first, I shall insist on several aspects which have been left in the dark until now.

Even if many of the institutions that were founded in the last sixty years have not really been associations *of* the disabled, but rather *for* the disabled, it would be misleading to claim that all these attempts were undertaken without the consent of the affected parties.[33] A number of these were the accomplishments of an ill or disabled person of great stature, both in France and abroad. Of course, these leading figures might gradually put a distance between themselves and real contact with new strata and new generations of the disabled, so that, in their turn, speaking on behalf of others . . . they are far from being recognized and authorized. This is one of the observations that one hears frequently among younger persons who have different requirements, claims very unlike their predecessors, images of themselves very distant from those of these pioneers. The generation gap, as in so many other domains. None of these disparities prevents us from claiming that the rich crop of institutions appeared with the consent of the persons concerned. The rehabilitation model was interiorized and is now anchored in the consciousness of the interested people. Disabled persons have demanded integration and have all along supported the direction taken by the associations. The disabled person's perception of self is a double image: an impaired being, and a citizen and worker like the others. Some small groups construct a new image for themselves and claim the right to "difference-within-equality" (there is currently a hint of dissidence, to which I shall return). But the great majority of people affected by the consequences of illness or accident adhere without hesitation to the idea of rehabilitation and, as a result, to that of the empirical normality of the social state of things (salaried industrial employment, living conditions, type of family, sexual norms, etc.).

The second point that I should like to make about the associations and other creations of all kinds concerns their evolution. Not all initially had the objective of rehabilitation or reintegration. But all institutions, whether they are (1) administered as specialized establishments, (2) for information or the exchange of opinions, (3) services for coordination, mutual assistance, and solidarity, or (4) organizations on the union model—*all* advertise that their purpose is to work for reintegration and rehabilitation. Even the associations for the mentally deficient.[34] The idea of rehabilitation henceforth polarizes all action undertaken on behalf of the disabled or, better, every action that calls itself social, for all aberrancy, from the amputation of a limb to delinquency is viewed, if not as curable (the first ambition), then at least as adjustable through control and regulation. From a certain perspective the plan for reintegration—and for rehabilitation—ended up dominating the idea of cure. A kind of realism, perhaps a cynical one, took over. Certain afflictions (paraplegia in the physical domain, schizophrenia in the mental domain, very low IQ in the cognitive domain, precocious deterioration in adjustment in the social domain) were considered as beyond recourse, as fundamental. But action could be initiated to alleviate the consequences of the affliction so that the individual might live normally. Recourse was had to technical aids, greater accessibility for the paraplegic, drug therapy for the mentally ill, work itself for the retarded, the guidance of social workers for the socially maladjusted, and so on. Once it had been recognized that we could (and should) rehabilitate and that we can scarcely hope to cure, a gradual shift occurred before our eyes in the idea of therapy and medicalization. The therapeutic agency—whatever the continuing significance of its power in its classical form[35]—is no longer principally the physician, but a collection of social workers among whom we see physicians gradually positioning themselves. In French the term *travailleur social,* "social worker," is still limited in its application to *assistants sociaux,* "social assistants," who for a long time were female, but the idea of a social intervention team composed of physician, psychologist, educator, and "social worker" in its strict sense is gaining ground. This evolution is notable because it marks the beginning of demedicalization that all analysts of the bureaucracy and the medical establishment (physicians and hospitals) have vigorously called for. But demedicalization is possible only through the intermediary of rehabilitation and reintegration. A new price must then be paid: the control and power of a collection of "intervenors" (*intervenants*), as the new phrasing has it. Power will be less concentrated—in the hands of the physician—and will be less visible, more devolved, even more elusive. This trend is also being strengthened by the counseling commissions (established by the law of 1975 in France), by the way in which "sectorization" is handled, and by some instances of decentralization, as in Quebec. The power claimed by these collectivities for social action is precisely to place, or leave, disabled persons in the ordinary social circuit, to merge them with the masses, to hide them in the very heart of the urban environment, to reduce distance, efface difference, give the appearances of normality. Specific rights are buried at the bottom of files opened only by the specialists; the illness or accident is guarded by medical confidentiality and the secrecy of commissions; control (even inequality) disappears into the streets walked by men and women all dressed the same.

Disability is to be as little apparent as possible, so that the rough spots on the social body remain unseen. Let's move to the common denominator, since the social networks that hold us, like wavelengths (so powerful) and electronic miniaturization (so active), can today be imperceptible. When visibility is sought, on TV screens, for example, it is not a network of multiple specialists that is shown but the disabled person living among all the rest. We need a detailed analysis of the visual and audio documents that are being produced today. In conferences as in the organizations, where films, photographs, and publications about the disabled are planned and realized, a consensus has been reached to avoid anything too specific: all gestures of pity are excluded but also all accentuation of disability and even more the social and administrative framing. Of course, when it becomes a question of extracting a few more bills from the public purse, they do not hesitate to turn the spotlight on a wheelchair, a drawn face, a family torn apart, an amputation. But when it is a question of showing "what society is doing" or how the disabled are situated within it, it is only and always normalcy that is represented.[36] Deficiency will always be concealed so that the image projected and retained by the spectator or auditor will be agreeable, not be aggressive, and, above all, not stigmatize any social wound. Our Western culture of the moment can no longer tolerate deformity. This fact leads us to seek out the hidden relationships that make this situation possible. But definitely not— and I cannot repeat this too often—to declare integration and fusion into this empirical normalcy a good thing or a bad thing. I do not say that normalization ought to be challenged; I say that it ought to be recognized for what it is.

The Word and the Thing or Nondistinction

In the year of this writing, 1997, I hesitate a great deal to revamp completely the text of the paragraph which follows. I finally opted to leave things as they were in 1982, because the essential was said then, even though it seems very useful to me to refer to my more recent work, cited in the footnotes.[37]

As we can all read, the word *handicap* from *hand-in-cap* passed from the vocabulary of gaming to that of horse-racing to designate an equalization of chances.

Many deplore that the idea of equal chances (primary sense) should be effaced by that of disadvantages (metonymical sense) in a transfer from the racetrack to human health. Few people think to question the moment and the conditions in which the word *handicap* appeared in French and replaced the word *infirmité.* Dictionaries only attest to the vogue of the word, parallel to the birth and development of rehabilitation.³⁸

The Robert dictionary, in its edition of 1957, calls attention to the figurative sense "to put in a position of inferiority" attested in 1889. In fact, the words *handicap* and *handicaper,* noun and verb, are found at the beginning of the century among authors to signify disfavor, hindrance (e.g., Bally, *Le Langage et la vie* [1913], 49; Gide, *Journal* [1924], 129, [1928], 50.) They are also found in the early work of Queneau, Céline, Vailland, but only in the 1920s and 1930s. The word *handicapé* as an adjective, on the other hand, is quite recent in French, and even more so as a noun to designate a disabled person. In contrast, *handicapage* and *handicapeur,* as racing and betting terms, have more or less disappeared and were never applied to the domain of disability or impairment. The Littré dictionary gives only the horse racing sense. A complete absence is to be noted in the Petit Larousse dictionary of 1906. The figurative meaning, "to constitute a disadvantage to someone," appears in the twentieth-century Larousse dictionary published in 1928. The eighth edition of the dictionary of the French Academy from 1932 also gives the figurative sense ("by extension, to be handicapped signifies to be put in a state of inferiority"). The *Larousse Encyclopédique* of 1962 gives only the extended meaning and not yet the specific meaning with reference to health. After the Robert of 1957, we have to wait until the 1968 supplement of the *Larousse Encyclopédique,* the Quillet dictionary of 1965, and all those that followed to find confirmed the narrower applications to medical, social, bodily, and mental matters. The law of November 23, 1957, introduced the word into legislative terminology ("is to be considered a handicapped worker . . . ," first article). The *Oxford English Dictionary* published a definition in which reciprocity figures plus the idea of an advantage given to the weakest of the horses:

> 1. The name of a kind of sport having an element of chance in it, in which one person challenged some article belonging to another, for which he offered something of his own in exchange. . . . 3. Any race or competition in which the chances of the competitors

are sought to be equalized by giving an advantage to the less efficient or imposing a disadvantage upon the more efficient. 4. The extra weight or other condition imposed upon a superior in favour of an inferior competitor in any athletic or other match; hence any encumbrance or disability that weighs upon effort and makes success more difficult. (1883)

In a single jump we have passed from a game of chance, the luck of the draw, and thus from a kind of natural fatality to a possible regulation, a will to master circumstance. A slight displacement of vocabulary and we have two different worlds in opposition: the world of disability, of insurmountable incapacity, and the world of handicap, of affliction compensated for. Pierre Oléron writes: "To speak of differences is to put the accent on what an individual lacks and is not capable of finding. A deficit is always present, a handicap that can be overcome" (*Bulletin de Psychologie* [January 1962]: 405). The handicapped person must recover his chances, chances equal to those of others. He should be able to compare himself to others; he should no longer be different, no more different than the horses that have been equalized. He should run the common course. This image of horse racing corresponds exactly to that of the handicapped person who has to catch up, rejoin the normal and normalized group, be one of them. The horse racing application of the word is the right one. *Handicap* as a designation of disadvantage, illness, amputation, loss is secondary in comparison to *handicap* signifying competition, rivalry, participation in a trial.

What is the current definition? The Petit Robert writes of *handicaper*: "to impose on a competitor some disadvantage according to the formula of handicapping." And for *handicap*, too, it writes of disadvantage, including in the figurative sense (a neologism, it adds), and for *handicaper*, figuratively, "disfavor, put in a state of inferiority." But these meanings of deficiency are results and do not indicate the linguistic evolution. This semantic shift occurred first in the application to bodily or social matters of what had earlier been used only of the racetrack. It will be rewarding to consider this definition in greater detail.

"To impose on a competitor some disadvantage . . ." Here we are dealing with constraint; he who intends a disadvantage for his competitor does so in the modality of obligation. What a terrible first confession: handicap presupposes a handicapper, who comes forward as a responsible controller. The recipient, for her part, is a "competitor," that is, subject to a program. A competitive program, a polemical program. The program is the choice of the handicapper alone. The competitors are identified as such independently of him; he only sets the "object" (the disadvantage) required for the realization of the program as conceived. Second avowal: the cause and the competition are givens, not up for discussion. The handicapper can act only on the handicap (the disadvantage) and owes his existence to it alone. The handicap is dysphoric, a disadvantage, a negative value.

The disadvantage is relative, "some disadvantage," that is, in horse racing it may be in terms of weight or distance and more generally anything that reduces performance. The word is open to considerable extension when it is transferred to the health or social domain. Every lessening of capability, of whatever kind, will be covered by the word *handicap*. It is a portmanteau word that permits indistinctness and thus confusion.

Let us continue the decryption of this definition, which now adds to the preceding elements: "according to the formula of handicapping." What had we learned about handicaps? "A disadvantage imposed on the better competitors so that chance are equalized." The ascription of disadvantage influences the running of the race: it gives equal *competence* to the competitors. But, clearly, using the word in the human sphere, handicap has become the diminution that lessens chances and it is the weakest who are handicapped. We will understand the semantic shift better when we recall that in horse-racing the disadvantage was imposed on the *strong* horses. Nonetheless, it is noteworthy that the definition of handicap introduces the equalization of competencies, and this is indeed the goal of rehabilitation. This linguistic juxtaposition is not by chance.

Four elements are then gathered: society is conceived of as a *competition*, almost a natural one; a handicap intervenes and imposes a supplementary burden: this burden is indefinite; the burden is overcome, and what was missing is restored. The word *infirme* (and all the words of deficiency in *in/im-*) does not carry this signification. Infirmity entails an exclusion, "out of the running." The French verb *infirmer*, which is not applied to the human world but only to things (like *invalider*) denotes a process of weakening. The use of *handicap*, *handicaper*, and *handicapé* is associated with a social will and context very different from those of the traditional words. Their appearance at the same time as the practice of rehabilitation marks a turning point in the way of addressing and treating disability.

It is no longer an almost radical difference that is designated, but *all* those who do not meet an ordained norm are categorized, in order to encourage them to recover it and reenter the competition of the industrial world and technological society. The introduction of new linguistic usage, with its denotations and connotations, contributes to society's collective representation of itself and also to its imaginings, at the same time as it is maintained by a style of life that can be described. Just what is this "lifestyle"?

The Courses to Be Run—Contradictions

Disabled persons, of all kinds, are henceforth handicapped, citizens thrown into the social competition, susceptible to reintegration. This presupposes and reinforces a society that sees itself as a normativized universal. I have analyzed this act of integration, clearly stated and yet new, as a decisive act toward understanding what has been happening since the start of this century. I understand it as an act of effacement, as an act of un-difference. In more than one way this last statement is shocking: from now on the disabled are often in the spotlight;[39] specific actions undertaken on their behalf are numerous; the general awareness of the interested parties is of an exclusion. I have tried to say to what extent the intention underlying legislation, the founders and their institutions, the terminology itself, was nonetheless expressive of a will to make disappear. The face of society should not have any pimples. "Would that we could all be the same!" Society's wish, as expressed through the treatment of disability, is to make identical, *without making equal.* In fact, measures and actions on behalf of impaired citizens tend to efface their difference but not establish them on the same level economically and socially. Of course, the racetrack vocabulary might encourage our social imagination to think that the chances had been equalized: the disadvantages of the "handicapped" are alleviated by therapies and compensatory training. But—and here we have to look closely—all these corrections and all these adjustments are intended primarily to facilitate reabsorption by the social body and only in very secondary fashion for valorization or advancement. The plan is not one of equality but one of identicalness. The gap between identity and equality is enormous. We are shaping a society that seeks the identical in inequality. While other societies have recognized difference in inequality, we hope for equality in difference. What are the courses to be run? Do they reveal this nonegalitarian culture of identicalness?

Labeling

We should note a flagrant contradiction, inscribed in administrative practice. We know that there is a recognition of disability in France, which is a product of the need to pass before specific agencies in order to enjoy the right to specific training or placement.[40] The disabled person then enters a category and carries a distinctive mark.

But it is not certain that the person in question may not already have been referenced and labeled before this measure. The purpose of this formal recognition is to facilitate the admission of the person into social and professional life. It's the passport. Paradoxically, it's an alien passport, for admission, finally, to be "like the others." After a certain time, or so it is claimed, the person is again socially suitable and qualified on the vocational level. Some people will go so far as to say that the disabled individual has to be overqualified. In other words, there is a labeling and the label is not removed (although the legislation does anticipate it) until the person is admitted to a "normal" employment situation where the disability must no longer count. This is the condition on which the individual finds a social place among the others. As I have already emphasized, the disability must no longer preclude anything, neither work, nor housing, nor public life. In short, disabled persons are admitted, readmitted as we say, if—and only if—the disability is no more than a secondary feature of the same order as height, hair color, or weight. The disabled person is integrated only when the disability is erased. Yet the mark follows him, just as it was imposed on him. We can say without exaggeration that the category of "disabled" is created and maintained, even when only the "formerly disabled," even the "dis-disabled," are integrated. A double constraint weighs on those in this situation: they are designated, pointed at, and pointed out (even in cases where there is no exterior physical sign) and they are expected to behave "as if nothing were wrong."

It would be fruitless to object, in the face of this analysis, that a whole series of amendments has been put in place, for example, the fact that in the business world the label remains because arrangements are required for working or salary conditions and, as much as possible, the quota of disabled workers must be met. As if this were not true for many others who are not labeled. In the final analysis the situation is this: a label stuck on a "normalization."

Here, then, is a society which is engaged in totemization, almost in the strict sense of Lévi-Strauss,[41] that is, distinguishing among social groups by means of a projection onto a series of exterior differences (here the horses on the racecourse), which at the same time calls for standardization. Moreover, this stage of almost indelible labeling is not imposed on all persons for the same reasons, even when there may be parity in the physical affliction. All those whose financial, cultural, and professional means permit the continuation or recovery of their prior integration are not affected by this labeling. Numerous observations made of the population admitted to specialized institutions establish the fact that only certain social strata are the object of the labeling process. Disability doubles the effect of some social situations, and not others. The deepest semantic value of handicap and disability is not medical but sociocultural.

Let us continue, for the moment, with the analysis of this label. There are also persons who bear the label but who have been identified as nonintegrable. These are individuals whose affliction has been called too serious. All kinds of special institutions have been created for them: MAS, group homes, sheltered workshops, nursing homes. Thus the general label of disabled is further subdivided into severe cases, mild cases, etc. The integration of some of these facilitates the recognition of others as unadaptable.

As concerns legislation, I have already insisted on the importance of naming. To name, designate, point out, is to make exist. Our natural assumption is to believe that language expresses the real, that it duplicates reality so that we can think about . . . and manipulate it, in our minds and in our conversations! But, quite to the contrary, language operates, transforms, creates. In one sense, there is no other reality than language. The institution of language is the primary social institution in which all the others are inscribed and, indeed, where they originate. This is doubtless the gain—and the principal gain—from what is called structuralism, and this is where the great writers of our generation come together, beyond their diverse and contradictory analyses or options. Not that language has a life of its own: such an expression is not adequate to the circumstances and makes one think of a biological organism. Language is an *institution,* in the double sense that it is socially established and that it arranges the social fact. Thus the phenomenon of the label *handicapé* is not just a bit of folklore: it is at the heart of the question. Establishing a general category that is further subdivided into offshoot nomenclature, society extends the fact of "handicap" as a consequence. This language grid allows every affliction to discover its correlates and to recognize itself, and permits every instance (medical or social) to pinpoint and steer. Control and direction are brought to bear on the slightest accident and on all kinds of illnesses.

Control of knowledge first of all, and this is the primordial role of the physician. The nomenclature in question is the possession of the doctor: he knows the language of etiologies. His act of naming is often without appeal: "She is . . . (myopathic, autistic, paraplegic), so what she needs is . . ." The doctor can *designate* and *classify.* In possession of this language, he can also lengthen or shorten the lists, put this or that individual on the list, take him off. We have seen the physician, almost a caricature, at the center of the initiative when it was time to post the obligatory quota of disabled (the law of 1957). According to circumstances and requirements, the labeling can be generous or restrictive. If necessary, a broken leg or missing little fingernail can be classed among disabilities or, inversely, a vocationally disqualifying illness is not on the list, just as circumstances dictate.

This practice has doubtless been modified by the provisions of the law of 1987. It would be of great interest to undertake a new inquiry of the relevant population: who is included in the quota?

The physician's language is rendered even more operative by the silences that he can exploit. This is medical secrecy. It is easy—and even respectable—to appeal to an elementary deontology. Each person has a right to confidentiality and it may be prejudicial that just anyone at all should gain access to one's medical file. But the medical secret is primarily a linguistic arrangement: to be able to speak or be able to keep silent. More powerful than the phrase, "She's a paraplegic, so that . . ." is this one: "I have to keep from you just what it is, but this is what we have to do. . . ." In the first case, the word names, and at time creates, pure and simple. In the second case, naming is eclipsed but something much more serious and dangerous is called into being . . . while knowledge is reserved for the physician. The language of the doctor here reaches an unparalleled sacralization. The God of the Old Testament, wishing to designate but not name himself and thus give unequaled mass to his unknown identity, had said, "I am who I am" (or, according to controversial translations, in an even more enigmatic formula: my name is "I am not nameable"). In the case before us it is a third party who has possession of the name and who transmits only the superficial designation of the secret. Here, in language, the physician assumes his supremely magical and religious role. In the social institution, he occupies the "divine" place. I earlier stated, in the chapter on the Jewish universe, that the priest was the sole authority to identify the presence of leprosy and that his verdict led to proscription. We can clearly see that this sacred, even sacrificial role of the priest has today passed to the doctor. [42]

Control over consequences. Picking up where the doctor leaves off is the series of social workers, the assimilators. The prior labeling permits and justifies the inquiry, the file. In order to declare a person disabled, measure the degree of the disability (required in order to allocate resources in appropriate degree), counsel this or that type of therapy program or establishment . . . the disabled person must become the object of discourse and a great deal of information then becomes necessary: emotional, family related, social, economic. And here comes the crowd of investigators: psychologist, social worker, representatives of la Tutelle (the governmental institution of public guardian), administrative secretariats. A crowd of agents works to formulate a language for the disabled. This discourse will permit selection: there are the disabled who can be reintegrated at little cost, there are those reintegrable under certain conditions, there are the "very severe" but still classifiable cases, and then there are the irretrievable (especially in the area of developmental retardation). This screening can offer paradoxes; I shall take just one example. Certain disabled persons, once the inquiries are finished and the commission has met, are subject to "direct placement," that is, someone judged that they could not complete vocational training or that they didn't need to. In both cases, it is proposed that they re-enter society . . . while looking for work. A whole long discourse has been realized to bring them to . . . the starting point. But from now on they are "disabled persons seeking employment" and will later be considered "disabled workers." These are certainly curious "reintegrables" (and reintegrated citizens): they have simply been rubber-stamped, which may be an advantage or disadvantage according to the case.

In addition to its screening function, the discourse required of the agents of social action allows detection upstream and tracking downstream. In order to give therapy and rehabilitation a maximum chance of success demands are made to address the illness or affliction as rapidly as possible, as close as possible to its moment of onset. In fact, the earlier an injury is cared for, the more easily it can be cured: common sense tells us so! The attention and concern of medical or social agents is then directed toward detection, toward locating cases. In France, this is actually made easier by sectorization, the existence of local health and social authorities. On the one hand, the body of information—and the exact label—allows (at least in principle, for an administrative compartmentalization is also at work) the disabled person to be accompanied and assisted as far as possible, or as she may herself wish. Maurice de la Sizeranne seems outdated when he declares that his association was to be a family for the blind from the cradle to the grave. But contemporary discourse also has a certain pretension toward a global mission. It is a discourse torn between specification (bordering on exclusion) and nondistinction (which thinks it tends toward integration).

This tug-of-war is still seen when different kinds of disability come into question. Two discourses arise. The one proposes to make careful distinctions among the kinds and classes of disability, the other to make the boundaries so fuzzy that there is scarcely more than a single class of the disabled.

The first discourse, by separating, makes it possible to prescribe particular measures that are adapted to each category. Let us take as an example the distinction between the physically and developmentally disabled. Common sense, you would say, indicates that we would not think to adopt the same medical techniques, that we would not envisage the same educational methods (basic schooling, upgrading prior knowledge, vocational training), that we would not, without insult and indignity, put these people in the same establishments. We would reason in the same way for social disability, psychological disability, etc. But is this the voice of difference? We note that the categories originate in a well-established "human geography": the body, intellect, psyche, social being. Within these large cultural categories, we are less scrupulous. Medical diagnoses and therapeutic resources make the difference; it is the same discourse that distinguishes the etiologies, but *in social terms* it knows of only a few large classes. In other words, I must call attention to a contradiction in this first kind of discourse: there is no desire to mix, but also none to differentiate below a certain level. Differentiation and specialization preoccupy society but at the same time society does not carry through on its impulse. There seem to be two logics: medical logic and social logic. Medical logic, still to a great extent clinical whatever people say, tends toward extreme social division. Social logic would willingly follow, provided that integration does not come to a halt. The desire is finally to integrate *all* the disabled, and the orientation of institutions for the developmentally disabled is the proof. But difficulties increase as this intention is applied to more and more cases and etiological classes. At the same time, the discourse of human geography of which I spoke makes it possible to limit this basic intention, while conserving it, and to continue the social division as long as uniformity is still not possible. On a more individual level, the discourse of limited distinction plays this same role, which could be compared to that of Janus: it makes it possible to reject certain disabilities (e.g., to deny the physically disabled reentry to the labor market, to deny the "retarded" hospital assistance) and to reaffirm adherence to the common discourse of reintegration.

I am conscious of the partial reversal of direction of this analysis in relation to others, well recognized. In fact, most often the relationship between the medical and the social is seen as follows: the doctors, belonging to the dominant strata of society, reflect the ideology of their class. In this relationship analyzed in terms of ideology, the medical is projected onto the social. But things seem more subtly set up to me, even the other way around. In fact, just as the social fact is easily subjected to psychological analysis today (e.g., power seen as enjoyment, conflicts interpreted as the rivalry of wishes or analyzed within the framework of a generalized Oedipus figure, etc.), so there is a projection of the medical onto the social. The significance of the medical is due not only to the status of physicians and medicine in society (which is nonetheless evident) but also to its own capacity for intervention and for knowledge. Society has been "etiologized." At the very same moment, the collected technologies—including medical technology—normalize, in conjunction with liberal political will (strongly identity oriented). The contradiction can be resolved in the "healing society." The true physician is the social worker or comparable agent, charged above all with reduction to the common denominator. In France we are accustomed to speak today of "health *and* social services."

The other discourse, while less frequent, is no less open to analysis. It shuffles the cards by claiming that the organic and the emotional are not separable, that the emotional and the social are linked, that the organic and the intellectual have something to do with one another. This discourse, too, takes its point of departure in a commonsensical recognition: you cannot lose a limb, or the capacity to walk, or your voice, or the faculty of speech without being affected, remade, dismantled in your psychological being. A good many studies have shown that there is a psycho-sociology of disability, of all disabilities. Just as there is a corporeality to all disabilities. The characteristic of this discourse is to reject the weaknesses of the other discourse, in the sense that it resists endless specialization, and thus institutionalization and separation by category. It is a militant discourse, and confrontational in one respect. But it is also a discourse close to that held by the representatives of public bodies and legislators (in France, particularly the legislators of 1975): enclose all forms of disability in a single embrace, deal with problems at once in order to give the appearance of a solution. This nondistinction is hardly very far removed from the distinction outlined earlier: in the first place because the labeling is the same, in the second place because the will to integrate is shown to be equally strong. It is not enough to have a slogan such as "disabled persons of all kinds, unite" to make the received category disappear. The category is so well established that we cannot speak today of any affliction without using the label "disability." There is consensus on the existence of disability.

As of the moment that a society assigns names, it is drawn toward the problem of integration. What everyone admits is the existence of disability. Some of the "disabled" raise the cry "disability doesn't exist,"[43] but this is only a slogan. Where, in social terms, does this widespread idea come from, that there are "disabilities"? Good sense will be heard, in the face of the impertinence—in all senses of the word—of the question. Physicians are certainly obliged to recognize the illness or accident that removes the individual from conventional conditions. And families certainly suffer enough when one of their members is not or who is no longer "like the rest." The state is certainly forced to take specific measures on behalf of citizens whose access to everyday life or work is denied. And yet the question may be asked. All deviation is defined in relation to a line, every abnormality in relation to a norm, every sickness in relation to an idea of wellness. There is no phenomenon that does not arise from history, and from social history. How does disability arise? Or, if you like, how does the phenomenon of the disabled arise? It arises from the fact that the environment, where the individual who suffers an illness or an accident lives, judges that it can no longer keep him. For example, the demands for necessary care cannot be met without the family separating itself from its member; or, possibly, the psychological burden in emotional terms is experienced as intolerable. Here, then, illness and accident refer to what the family is, in its social context. Business, to take another example, experiences an incompatibility between its objectives—principally profit—and the impaired salaried employee. But here, as well, the problem is one of modern business. Or the hospital that has cared for a person for a certain time can neither send her home nor keep her. She has to be handed over to different but still specialized institutions. For the third time, our interrogation comes to bear on the medical system and hospitalization.

It is not my intention to develop an analysis of the contemporary family, business, and medicalization. I simply want to recognize that labels and categorization originate in social structures much more than in the simple fact of physical and psychological affliction. In our Western society, the desire to integrate rises out of the incapacity of the social fabric to permit the disabled person to live there. I repeat that it is not for the moment a question of making value judgments or of saying whether things can be done in a different way. The disabled are becoming more and more numerous, not by reason of sicknesses or accidents which might be increasing (the progress of medicine that saves or lengthens life, the appearance of new diseases, increased risk of accidents at work, etc.), but because the basic social fabric will less and less preserve the affected individual and will label more and more people. Society can take supplementary measures of the curative, even preventative, type, but the problem is not there. It is on the level of what leads to designation. It is the obligation in which society finds itself to attribute the qualifier *disabled* that creates the disability socially. This constraint itself comes from the organization of sociability. Any distance from very strict and narrow norms (the single-family model, nuclear and centripetal, the requirements of schooling, the production imperative, the excess of medicalization) will become less and less admissible. And it can't be a few lucid statements to make clear the distinction between maladjustment and disability that will reverse the process. The margin of acceptance for every aberrancy is retracting to the extent that the imperatives of groups who establish sociability become more precise and more rigorous. In our society *disabled* will increasingly be synonymous with *maladjusted.*

Every failure to adjust will be labeled a disability. We are caught in a process that is almost insane: the least maladjustment will be cataloged, referenced, and made into a disability, which will in turn entail specific measures, even initiate some very specialized programs before deficient adjustment is declared normalizable. If we take into account elderly persons especially, we could almost say that the vast majority of the population will be disabled, with the social norm taking refuge in a small number of individuals. This normal individual will preferentially be white, male, young, healthy, handsome, educated, and . . . submissive!

The contradiction is startling: labeling produces the disability and is producing more and more. Labeling is there to facilitate access to a process of normalization! This is why the thesis of exclusion has its rationale: maladjustments are increasing, tracking and identifying are becoming more refined, the solutions are decreasing in number! The thesis of the "will to integrate" that is advanced here cannot be simplistic. But the label is not the sole means employed by our society in the face of disability.

Subsidizing

Track and name. Once this is done, a series of actions must be initiated to reduce the disability and make integration possible. And each one of these actions depends on one factor: money. What is being paid for? Who is paying? How is payment effected? This last is an important question for understanding the rehabilitation issue, which is entirely dependent on funds that are allocated or withheld.

I have already stated that the expansion of institutions and resources for rehabilitation and retraining dates from the legislation of 1945 dealing with social security. Rehabilitation took off when it could be funded. A labeled person has real and specific rights only when some jurisdiction assumes responsibility for covering the costs incurred (*la prise en charge*). The case can be the object of a program as soon as the financial aspect is determined. The French phrase makes it clear that this funding is not directed to the person in question but is a reimbursement for costs incurred by the person. In Western systems of social security it is never a question of direct subsidies to the citizens, but of sparing them the costs of the services that have been seen as necessary. These services have to be recognized as such: it is the doctor's prescription, the obligatory hospitalization, the recognized status as disabled worker, etc. It is the *medical* decision that activates rights for the payment of services. In the same way that the doctor's prescription is the reimbursement stub for the consultation and medication, it is the fact of being recognized as "disabled" to such and such a degree that constitutes the voucher for the coverage of the more or less substantial costs entailed by entry into a specialized institution.

In the overall social budget for disability (154 billion francs in 1992 [US$ 25 billion]) cash benefits are the largest component at 73 percent; benefits in kind represent only 27 percent. This does not prevent my observation that the costs of institutionalization continue to be high. Subsidy remains one of the preferred means of funding. But above all it is important to note that the money is divided among benefits and institutions, but little goes to direct human aid, to social workers who would have the task of creating sociability, an ordinary social environment around people. In other words, nothing is paid so that civil society might be supported, stimulated, incited, assisted in living with disabled persons. It's not a question here of making a case for or against these benefits and institutional cost coverage. It is nonetheless remarkable that nothing that could make a strong contribution toward the presence of the impaired among the others is ever a budget line item.[44]

In Western countries the complex of financial aid systems intersect one another. In France there is essentially one kind of financial benefit for disabled adults (who do not work), which can be accompanied by subsidized housing and a compensation grant (that is, a "third-person" grant or one for supplementary costs incurred by employment). For children the chief benefit is special education, which is a family grant and which may also have certain supplements. As concerns revenue, for adults who work there is also a system of "guaranteed income," determined in relation to the guaranteed minimum wage in which any discrepancy between the salary and the minimum wage is made up by the state in the form of a complementary payment.

To these essential arrangements must be added old age security for mothers who have a disabled person at home; disability identity card, good for transportation and the reduction of certain other expenses; some scholarships; some financial aid to employers to adapt work stations, for the training of disabled apprentices; some bonuses associated with redeployment. Finally and in particular, vocational trainees (in the process of redeployment) receive a salary based on the guaranteed minimum wage or on their prior salary. Despite the apparent abundance of these subsidies, such financial assistance often does not amount to an income higher than the guaranteed minimum—except during the period of vocational training, when there is coverage of expenses and remuneration. And despite this apparent abundance, the essential outlay remains the assumption of costs for institutional stays (for care or training).

Before, in trade and barter, the inequality of lots or of the objects exchanged was compensated for: this was the adjustment. This compensation has given way, as concerns disability, to the subsidy. If we consider the grants made directly to the persons affected, they have a name: *allocations* (benefits). The word *allocation* does not have an exact orientation and in its primary signification it refers to a grant of money. Such grants have their own history. They are connected with the subsidies made to the family. They were initially bonus payments, then public compensation for family responsibilities (with a variety of objectives: psychological, demographic, preventive). They were reduced in France during the 1950s and were made dependent on income at the end of the 1960s (with a reduction in the number of beneficiaries). In short, benefits went from being nearly identical with social security grants based on cross-subsidization, with the redistribution favoring low family incomes, to a tendency to resemble public aid as it was conceived of by the nineteenth century.[45] This is a system focused on detail that misunderstands the general problems of social life and places categories that are already disadvantaged in a position of isolation, a form of ghettoization. The essential point of this analysis is that these benefits—whose quantity is not a real problem since the

Western countries are wealthy, even in moments of crisis[46]—can re-place all other efforts on behalf of the disabled. It is easy to assign labels. It is easy to pay—but just a little at a time—to the extent this is all that is asked. On the model of "Be beautiful and keep quiet" we have "Take your benefits and don't ask for more." People will pay as much as needed—in the double form of subsidies to institutions and aid to individuals—in order to make the problems of social misery disappear, in the desire to leave the social surface as it is and without necessarily reducing inequalities.

Paying seems easier than establishing aggressive programs to off-set the problems of these deficiencies. This is paradoxical, it would seem, when we know that social policy is moving to second rank in importance and that social budgets are always restrictive and quite disproportionate in relation to others, for example, the military bud-get. And yet, at the very core of social work, preference is readily accorded to benefits rather than to vocational training and therapy. The latter are expensive in the short term but we can expect of them a lessening in the need for benefits in the long term. A person put back to work becomes productive again, pays taxes, and no longer receives benefits. The preference for benefits is not a simple question of close-fisted financial calculation. It seems to me that monetary assistance makes it possible to forget disability. The business community, caught up in keen competition and the race for profits, doesn't want to see disabled persons in their "temples."

A kind of incompatibility is created between this neosacral space and the profane character that a deformed, that is, simply dissimilar, body or mind assumes. It is clear, here as in many other points in this book, that we cannot deny all the efforts and attempts in the opposite direction. There are various organizations, groups of employers, official regulations that give priority to complete reintegration over monetary payments. The contradiction is everywhere present in our Western societies. But there remains an irreconcilable element in the relation-ship between *industrialized* society and the impaired.

It is not impossible that we have here a substitution phenomenon: paying in order to make the disabled person disappear is a form of killing. But this "sacrifice" no longer has anything to do with a real sacrifice. It is a social death. From every point of view, our societies have found the means, or at least have sought them, to erase aberrancy. The will toward integration, including in work and in salaried employment, that I have emphasized so much, is contemporary with this incompatibility. Another matter is what gives society its global structure, another matter, too, all the kinds of resistance that try to oppose it. Society never advances at a uniform pace, and several anthropologies are at work at the same time.

The issue here is the will, wide-spread and widely shared, to make difference socially invisible. In many respects, to the benefit of those concerned, I admit: it is not a question of denigrating the hope to enjoy life like everyone else. This wish must be fully honored. But in seeking out what is still hidden behind the social act of an integration that would deny difference, we have a chance of not simply buying into public demands. Paying, paying in the double form of subsidy and aid, preferring to pay in certain cases rather than to integrate in certain places, seems to my eyes a reinforcement of this social death of the "differing body." The exclusion of old is finished; what replaces it is an assimilation, an assimilation, and thus a new form of pulverization. The kinds of exclusion which remain—numerous as they are—are only the other side of this technocracy of absorption.[47]

Rehabilitating

Caring   The medical eye is everywhere. An immense power, which has taken up where father confessors and *directeurs de conscience* (spiritual advisors) left off. The proof no longer needs to be laid out, so numerous are the analyses. But the analyses clearly have not changed anything: this power is still in place and holding firm.[48] The dimensions of this power have been stated time and time again: exclusive possession of knowledge, limitation of access to information and medical "secrets," the position as "counselor" and social "monitor" (e.g., through the division into administrative sectors, which replaces the space of the asylum without surrendering control over the "insane"), etc. The power network of physicians and medicine is tight, intense, far-reaching. I shall not rehearse the analysis of this network at present. I shall address the role of the doctor in her capacity as therapist, where she enters the process of therapy. What is there to say?

Physical therapy consists of restoring the individual to the same freedom of movement and action as previously, to the greatest extent possible. Mental, educational, emotional, and social therapy equally well consist of recovering earlier capacities and knowledge, even of enhancing them. But assuming the role of therapist presupposes setting up a relationship of master to pupil and giving priority to one project over another. Considering the French term for therapy (*ré-éducation*) in its etymological sense (from Latin *e-ducere*, "to lead out from the subject itself"), we see that there is scarcely any true neutral therapy. When care calls itself therapy, the physician is already much more than a physician. This can be clearly seen because everywhere within the universe called "rehabilitation" the physician is the principal actor in counseling the impaired person. He makes pronouncements on the level of therapy, of course, but also on the level of the desirable follow-up to his own actions: he is present, at the heart of all the instances that will determine the fate of the disabled person[49] and thus the rights that will be accorded him. It is common knowledge that the physician's advice—especially when accompanied by the famous medical secrecy—weighs heaviest.

Care is more than just caring for. The link between rehabilitation institutions and services, and medicine is so strong that it is not possible to dissociate their involvement over the last fifty years. The pioneers of physical medicine, of therapeutic medicine[50] had the following simple idea: what is the good of restoring to someone a certain control over her body if nothing or no-one restores her to a condition in which she can learn, work, and live among others? But, in so doing, the physician also sets himself up as an agent of rehabilitation, even in cases where he intended to "hand the case over" to instructors, vocational therapists, psychologists, etc. Care becomes an all-encompassing action. Attendance at conferences, study days, colloquia of all kinds, quite frequent in the world of rehabilitation, make this all too clear: the physician is positioned as one of the speakers on rehabilitation and as such speaks very little of medicine in its narrow sense.

This analysis confirms the analysis of the medical authorities.

But I would like to insist on one very particular aspect of this power—if we continue to use this word to designate the ramifications of the decisive influence of doctors. Official arrangements ascribe to physicians—in structural terms—an educational, formative function. This lends weight to the idea that the *res publica,* including the state, has a nurturing character. Public instances, here especially the administrative, no longer conceive of themselves as simple services of facilitation and coordination, but as charged with an anthropological task. This is not an original observation: it has been known since the nationalization of schools, for example. But it shows how extensive this is. And here we can see that, despite the words, therapy and rehabilitation are not that far apart, because therapy under public control has no other goal than further adaptation to society and to its more or less diffuse models. Even if, as I said earlier, the medical and social elements are not to be seen in a relationship where the latter simply reflects the former, nonetheless therapeutic medicine— the sense of which is wider than the activity of healing—constitutes one of the intermediaries of this social adaptation. I am not saying that we could do otherwise with the social framework that we have; how could governmental departments, for example, not attempt to establish a close link between training systems and the needs of industry? But this should not obscure the fact that our whole present-day society is constricted and obsessed by social conformity. Society must recognize this if it is to survive its own actions.

If medicine assumes this role of therapist, it is also by reason of its relationship to the body, and not only to society. And it would be harmful to claim, in simplistic fashion, that the one is dependent on the other. What is the medical view of the disabled body? Does this view differ from the current medical view of the sick body? The medical viewpoint has been analyzed many times over.[51] The view of the therapy specialist is no doubt marked by great humanism, since it has its origins in a concern for humankind and in personalized circumstances, and struggled for forty years to break free of the perspective of the clinic (Foucault). It is situated less in the monitoring register than in that of training. This is not to say that features of the asylum—

especially important for insanity—do not exist in the sphere of disability: there are many specialized hospitals on the model of psychiatric hospitals where, in the calm of this therapeutic isolation space, the physician observes, classifies, treats, as if it were a question of selected plants, as if it were a question of sicknesses accidentally carried by the sick. Specialization exists, with its inevitable tendency toward internment and medical abstraction. But the medicine that is called therapeutic has not gone very far in this direction. Despite the highly concentrated numbers,[52] the spirit of this medicine is closer to that which launched the division into sectors than to the old spirit of the asylum.[53] A concern for a certain global dimension on the one hand, a focus on integration into life and work environments on the other alleviated the rigor of the asylum for the mentally ill, even for the developmentally impaired. In addition, there was never a law for the developmentally impaired parallel to that of 1838, just as there was no correspondence to the circular letter of 1960 that established this sector.

The medical view of the disabled evolved as more paternalistic than clinical, more concerned with training than healing. The connection with the sick body is not the same for the simple reason that there is often no healing. And here, in contrast to the psychiatric domain, no illusions are possible: the man or woman in a wheelchair, using crutches or other devices, is a *visible* fact. There are compensations, rectifications, replacements, either through surgical means or through long-term treatment,[54] but there is no suppression of the malformation as such. It is inevitable that recourse is had to therapy. The sick body is to be straightened up but not to be cured. Henceforth, the difference in the way of looking at another's body and an other body is obvious. Above all, it becomes necessary to reduce the effects of the illness or impairing accident. It is a fairly easy move then to the art of hiding these effects to the greatest extent possible (which is, in any case, demanded). The role slips from the strictly medical area to a more general role as life counselor. Here the physician is at his closest point of resemblance to other social workers. This is equally true of the front-rank position that genetic illness has assumed. If we except the researchers who are at work on the human genome project, the doctors in contact with the public constitute a mixture of physician and social counselor.

Training and "Shaping Up"

Therapy, understood as a project effected on the disabled person and as a normalization, is not the physician's action alone. Afterwards, training (Fr. *formation*) takes over. I am not speaking here of schooling, which is the lot of all children, because I am not trying to analyze the relationship between our society and its desire to instruct.[55] Training is something else. If the French word *formation* has been used rather vaguely to designate all instructional activity, it has been particularly associated with employment in the phrase *formation professionnelle* (vocational training). To meet the needs of industrial production and in association with technological change, a beginning was made in the last century to develop an educational mode that was not aimed at cultural development, at a general humanist level, but at the acquisition of knowledge and attitudes that were adapted to jobs in production. The French term *former* (both *shape* and *train*) was then being applied in its stricter sense: to place in a mold, shape in a certain way, cause the worker to exist by arranging him, conceiving of him in a certain way. Now one of the important aspects of rehabilitation—in the principal European countries—was to conceive and create a system for training, in particular vocational training.[56] All these various kinds of training aim at the creation of a disabled worker, adapted to the world of production and playing the role of salaried employee. In training of this kind, the idea of rehabilitation is present, but the project is a more precise one: rehabilitation for industrial work.[57] This is why there is a certain number of social roles next to the physician as rehabilitator. For example, the work psychologist, a title that is transparent: it is really a matter of seeing when, how, and under what conditions an individual will be able to enter the production system, ought to enter it, will enter it . . . or stay in it.

This function, little known to the general public, is positioned at very strategic points along the path of the disabled person: at the moment of general counseling, at the moment of entry into one of the processes that is to assure her integration. Another important role is that of the *moniteur technique* (vocational rehabilitation supervisor); again, the name is significant. Often the product of industry, himself "formed" in an apparatus whose entire conception has as an objective its adaptation to business,[58] the supervisor has been put in place to effect social "reproduction," according to the concept made popular by the work of P. Bourdieu and J. Passeron. Finally, there is a third person in this training process: the social assistant. Charged with the work of detailed knowledge (of the situation of the individuals affected on the one hand, of the sociojuridical framework on the other), she plays the role of placement officer. In actual fact, the social worker determines where the disabled worker is best placed—and best aided by personalized assistance to keep that place.

A society cannot live with a consciousness of its deepest motivations, any more than you can speak a language while being conscious of all the grammatical rules to which you are subject.

There is yet another person that should be mentioned, who plays different roles according to the rehabilitation sector in question: this is the *éducateur* (training specialist). In the vocational training sector he does not have a role of the first rank. A supplement, stand-by, complement, if you like, but he is not a major player. Moreover, many vocational rehabilitation and training institutions do without this function. When he does exist, he is asked principally to contribute to, not to contravene, the adjustment of the disabled to society and to the society of labor.

In contrast, in other sectors, those of children and in particular of maladjusted or troubled youth, these functionaries play an important role. This is understandable, since it is a question of preparatory phases prior to social and vocational rehabilitation. They are then the principal, indeed the only, agents. But from them, too, a reintegrating activity is expected. This often provokes crisis and tension because, from their perspective and by choice, they are particularly sensitive to the differences among their trainees, and are ill at ease in the social function of educating and training people *for* something. The contradictions of the system are apparent here, but so is its principal structure. We produce specialists for many training programs and sensitize them to individuals and to specific conditions, but on the social level we expect them to contribute to an action to restore people to the norm. The education, recruitment, working conditions, salaries of trainers—all put them at the painful crossroads of rehabilitation: they are expected to go and find, and understand, difference in order to fit it back into the established canon. Often the trainers, worn out with this tug-of-war, give up or frequently cross the line to become in their turn the heads of institutions, psychologists, or social workers.

Here we can give a negative demonstration of the will to train the disabled, that is, to adapt them to the production process. There is, we know, a formula called the sheltered workshop. The person who, in the minds of the diagnosticians and instructors, cannot go into the business world or undergo the vocational training that would provide access to it is offered industrial work in special shops where the pace, type, and conditions of productivity have been lowered and adapted. This is the working environment for a great number of the developmentally retarded. The sheltered shop is an asylum-like workhouse, where one could spend one's entire life, and is defined by the impossibility of integrating the industrial labor environment: the proof that social aspirations are focused on wage earners. These protected enclaves exist only by means of sub-contracting for normal businesses: an entrepreneurial pose, more or less successfully pulled off. I am not saying whether this is the lesser of two evils, or not. I only want to say that, from the social perspective these are inferior forms of industrial work. This is common knowledge. They are still a way of integrating, although it may appear exclusion. I prefer to see them as aborted forms of a more complete integration, for in the discourse of disability this is the way they are spoken of: a way of approximating the worker's status when other routes have shown themselves to be impossible.

Thus, exclusion is only the reverse side of one kind of inclusion. The latter remains the goal. Paradoxically, we can say that it is here that the training policy reaches its zenith: people wholly riveted to their production task. Here I see why vocational training was not developed from within these employment structures. Such training is designed to adapt the worker to her task; if she can be adapted without such instruction, it is even more of a success. The question of disability then reveals quite clearly the exact meaning of the *formation,* "training," that society intends to promote on behalf of its citizens. Moreover, whoever breaks the rules risks being reduced to social misery. There is no room, even for one whose body or mind is different, for anything but the tasks assigned by production.

What I am stating here does not contradict what I said earlier about the rejection of the disabled from the world of industrial labor. There is a tension, a contradiction. Sheltered employment, by its intermediate character, drives a wedge between ordinary work and segregation, and perfectly illustrates the situation where the detour—therapeutic, educational, or simply a waiting period—becomes a one-way street without return. Integration is the objective, but the action cannot be completed, and the persons affected remain in a liminal state.[59]

Mixed Schemes and Principles
of Redistribution

So far, I have hardly gone beyond simple description. This was necessary in order to give some weight to this exposition, already quite elaborated, because we are not dealing with a documentary photograph. Assuming the anthropologist's stance, I am trying to see what happened when present-day Western society encountered disability. In doing this, I seek both to illuminate the situation of the disabled and to understand—on the basis of this limited but quite exemplary instance—this society. This task is more difficult than for societies that are distant from us. The most difficult thing to understand is what we, ourselves, are engaged in. This insurmountable historical condition may cause some people to renounce the analysis of their own society. This is customarily the ethnologist's attitude, as it is the historian's. The sociologist often makes a greater attempt to investigate the present. Perhaps, ultimately, it is still the one who cracks the code of systems that "make sense" who is least poorly placed to undertake this risky adventure. This is where the gamble occurs, at least in part. It does have the advantage of not taking on society in its entirety but of

entering surreptitiously by a small door. The problem of disability is a
bit like the shard of pottery discovered during an archaeological dig
that justifies important observations on the culture of which it is the
vestige. To change our imagery, it is a bit like the cliff-side view over a
whole valley or the obstacle that tests the condition of the athlete or,
finally, the barometric reading that tells us the weather.

The moment has then come to try to reconstruct a bit of our culture, on the basis of these fragments. First of all, there is our heritage,
the program of charity. We inherit this from the nineteenth century but
also from the distant past of Christianity. Still to be written is the history
of "charity," which was not always the same phenomenon over the
course of centuries (here the work of Lallemand is certainly not adequate). Without any doubt, at the outset the creation of institutions had
the character of good works as they had earlier existed. This can be seen
in several respects: all began with benevolent intentions, appealing for
contributions, taking collections, receiving legacies. All were supported by individuals' feelings of piety and guilt. All took the attitude—
even while making claims for their inherent dignity—of submission to,
and collaboration and negotiation with, public and governmental powers. These characteristic features are referable to the ideas of replacement, compensation, and remediation that governed charitable works.
In addition, assistance, although without ambition as concerned equality, was still part of people's thinking. Finally, "willpower" was in fashion: the first necessity was to *want to do well*, do all that one could, have
a passion to compete with the able, never give in . . . and never falter or
despair. The institutions that were created then addressed themselves
to inner forces, to the power of the will. Will, the primary modality of
action, reigned over the period of institutional foundations. This appeal
to willpower—which also screened out the good disabled from the less
good or poor—is quite closely linked to the program of charity as it was
inherited from the past: assistance was based on merit on the one hand,
and should have no pretension to be critical of political reasoning on the
other. We can add another, much less obvious element to the register of
charity. Christian history had elevated charity into a universal (since,
fundamentally, it came from God and belonged to him).[60] Charity, even
when understood in sociological terms and no longer in a theological

perspective, appears as the superior value and soon afterwards as the remedy, the supreme solution, always sufficient, necessary, and effective. Charity—yet again, and even when cut back and ideologically broadened—was conceived of as sufficient and not only as necessary.

But this first scheme was challenged by others and lost its dominance. Ideas of rights, of social reparation, of redistributive justice had appeared. I have noted this in the case of the victims of war or work-related accidents. Also, in the domain of disability we soon see appear comparable demands, accompanied by a call for charitable conduct. The ethical, and even political, universals meet head on, but balance each other out. Charity, the founding principle of ethical and social order for centuries, endures but becomes tangled among other ideas issuing either from the struggle of the exploited classes or from economic and technical development (the idea of assimilation to the community of the normal). To the extent that the idea of charity persists, it directs a series of practices, such as the appeal to a philanthropic attitude, devotion to an almost spiritual mission, fear of opposition to government power. In the disinterested service of a form of poverty the worker at rehabilitation institutions had the dominant characteristic of being an "apostle" before being a professional, of being generous before being salaried, a kind of lay brother or sister, marked in the first hand by a sense of vocation. And this corps of social workers, in all logic, could not make claims against a government that was itself viewed in "charitable" optics (by citizens as intermediaries) and never critically seen as a manipulator of economic or ideological interests. Thus, the institutions were content with weak resources, very loose coordination, and minimal rationality. These tendencies resulted not only in the present geography of rehabilitation but also in the funding system, in an incapacity to coordinate efforts in an organic and efficient way,[61] in lax administrations, in the recruitment of personnel according only to moral criteria.

But since the idea of charity was overturned by new programs, certain rehabilitation institutions were taken over by social organizations (trade unions, health insurance funds, activist movements). This happened fairly late, after World War II. But even before, a more collective view, based in rights and the need for solidarity, had

appeared to compensate for the limitations of the charity system.[62] At
the very beginnings of rehabilitation, issues deriving from liberalism
were added to the program of charity, even in this moderated form.
The collusion between bourgeois liberalism and rehabilitation is neither simple nor mechanical in its action. The liberal element enters
the system, contributes to it and in so doing adapts itself so as to
recreate the system and stay within it. This observation is also of
general relevance: when a system of thought and action gets a foot-
hold, it assimilates various prior elements but does not leave them
intact. To underline this aspect is not just to admit a simply shaded
analysis, it also shows what constitutes a system, how and *under what
conditions* a system is constituted.

The liberal element that penetrated the rehabilitation system
seems to me what I would call a naturalism of the artificial. There is no
need today to recall that liberalism, in its fundamental guise, is content to await both economic development and social harmony from the
spontaneous engagement of individual initiatives. We also know very
well that this liberalism had been able to adapt wonderfully well to the
very strong demands of long-range governmental planning and to au-
thoritarian intervention. With the double weapon of confidence in the
regulatory interplay of interests and the cult of willpower in order to
prevent an imbalance among established interests, liberalism is a
prodigious assimilator of new policies, which it allows to emerge and
even grow only to subordinate them finally to the preestablished system. The appearance of rehabilitation can serve as example. The liberalism that was heir to the nineteenth century was convinced of the
necessity to assist, even with large-scale, specialized means. The form
of remedy that rehabilitation offered was *curative* and *reintegrating.*
In other words, rehabilitation did not initially address the social and
economic causes and conditions which gave rise to disability, no more
than it questioned itself on the final outcomes of this society. The
inherent naturalism of liberal thought consists in seeing all forms of
impairment as accidents; it is no one's fault when someone inadver-
tently falls from a ladder. To move this idea to the level of society:
there are accidents just as there are illnesses; these things happen,
happen inevitably. It is necessary to heal and to reintegrate; there is no

question of preventing this from happening. Nor is there a question of turning back to *where all this happens.* The whole company of rehabilitation pioneers (who were contemporary with the great social and economic analyses that had been made possible by the masters of the preceding century) all accepted this neonaturalism with regard to society. Reinforcing the belief that, faced with sickness and disability, one can only heal, restore, compensate, but not at all avoid, liberal society convinced itself that there was nothing to be done about accidents due to the dangers of technological society (work, wars, speed, etc.). The supreme accomplishment was to propose to the person who was victim of these economic arrangements to come back and participate in this society, just as before and like the others. The means were not lacking for this course of action. Once liberalism saw the advantage it could draw from the situation (the untouchability of the established order), it gave a great deal, or rather encouraged a great deal. A very concrete example may be shown: medicine caused the retreat, even the disappearance, of certain diseases (here, liberalism is preventive . . . in an indirect way) such as tuberculosis—which was the major preoccupation between the two wars and until the end of the 1950s—or poliomyelitis, which was conquered through vaccination from 1962 onward. During this decrease, other afflictions grew in number and kind, due to accidents at work and in traffic or, like nervous depression and psychosis, aggravated by the conditions of modern life. What did they do? The old tuberculosis "sans" were transformed into centers for functional or vocational rehabilitation and the psychiatric hospitals filled up and multiplied in number. There was a rush to the new populations of the disabled; the establishment of new facilities or the adoption of new methods of treatment were accelerated. But no policy of prevention was drafted, no more than decisions concerning the modality of life (the automobile, for example) were envisaged. The rehabilitation centers act as if many disabilities have an inevitable character. The artificial side of industrial society, its mode and capacity to produce, consume, sell, takes on a quality of the natural, of something that goes without saying, that one cannot seek to change without posing a threat. The whole construction of industrial liberalism makes it out to be the most natural thing in the world, the product of good sense, of harmony, of health . . . and, to top it all off, of happiness. Its conditions, and thus its grave threat to the physical and psychological integrity of many persons are also presented as natural features.

But the liberalism from which rehabilitation was crafted did not stop at this liberalism of the artificial. It had at its disposal powerful resources as a consequence of technological development. It would then fight back against disease or the consequences of accident; its naturalism is not the fatalism of the ancients. It is inevitable that accidents occur, part of the natural order of a developed society, but it is not inevitable that the consequences remain untouched; such is the technological order of this same society. With its bases and from its inception, liberalism presented itself as immutable. With its potential for evolution and conquest, it cloaked itself in change and progress. Playing on both dimensions, it gave itself an impressive permanence. Disability cannot be avoided, but it can be compensated for in better and better ways: the science of effacement, of forgetting, of restoration does exist.

This—unspoken—discourse of liberalism was never projected as such by the founders of and foundations for rehabilitation. But we know that discourse does not have to be uttered explicitly for it to inform praxis. For my purposes, here, I will take the example of the silences that punctuate the discourse of the founders and foundations that I am speaking about. In the two decades between the wars, texts on the suffering of the disabled, on the personal assumption of illness and disability, on the drama of families, on the individual resources that a human being has to overcome disadvantage . . . these texts appeared by the hundreds, thousands. I have found none that poses the problem of the roots of disability in the type of society we have, in other words, that addresses the prejudgment and thus the prejudice of the inevitable character of the production of certain disabilities.

We would make a great mistake to think that this summary analysis of the survival of an idea of charity, now become inadequate and mixed into a liberal, bourgeois vision, constituted some kind of primal, a priori scheme of things. I refer to the double historical origin of the concept of rehabilitation. But we must realize that we are facing a divided vision, and thus a cultural scheme that goes far beyond any single social class or stratum. What directs the position that I call charity is the idea of compensation by means of remediation. This idea is so taken for granted that I have never seen anyone propose to change fundamentally this way of situating the problem. What matters is the means by which the disabled will be put on a par with the others, understood of course as the able-bodied. What differentiates a narrow conception of charity and the expanded notion of which I am speaking is a strategy: those who hold the first view do not want to confront the authorities and they expect the essential to come from the kind hearts of individuals. Those who hold the second view are aware of structural inequalities and demand collective remedies. In both cases, it is a matter of reducing the distance between those held back and those in advance. Of a society *inherently differentiated,* for example, there is no question. The thing that is the most generalized and mentally shared is once again confirmed: reintegrate, that is, assimilate and, to do this, offer the steps most suitable to saddle one's handicap successfully, to return to the racetrack where the concept of handicap originated.

As for the liberal idea of the inevitable, random, and natural character of disability, it may seem that it belongs to a social class. But it should be noted that the very persons who attribute disability, at least certain disabilities or the penalties of disability, to society, are engaging in a kind of sociological naturalism: it is society that produces the disabling character of disability. It is difficult to argue with this claim, whichever way you turn it, on such a general level. But everyone admits that society today could not be otherwise than industrial, economically expansive, divided into social classes, productive,[63] thus other than a fabricator of disability. It is true that some people call for a society that is different from that organized by liberal and capitalist thought. In this sense, disability is not being made into social destiny. But, unless there is proof to the contrary, I cannot see that there is a significant reduction in the social causes of disability in countries where the principles of the liberal bourgeoisie do not rule. Nor does one see develop, in these cultural zones, a nonsociological way of thinking about disability. You may protest at what seems an awkward effort to reduce what is essentially a historical train of thought—such as Marxism—to a neonaturalism, even to a form like that of liberalism. This is not what I am saying. I simply want to say that we cannot so easily exorcize the idea of a fated inequality and above all the idea, relevant to my topic, of a certain common order where difference is supposed to disappear. Let's look at things the other way around from what I have just said. In its aims, ideological but also real, liberal thought envisages progress, including social progress. From certain economic developments are to be expected a reduction in inequalities, or at least a harmony that would no longer be perceived as inegalitarian. Liberal naturalism is as if compensated by its indestructible faith in technology. By considering this view as the very example of an ideology and by putting social development on another base, progressive sociological thought—of the Marxist kind in particular—nonetheless subscribes to a conception of history, by way of the very notion of progress, that reduces inequalities but *also* differences. Moreover, it is not for a simple, superficial reason of tactics or even of strategy that the great social forces, such as the parties on the left, in particular those of a Leninist bent, back off from a struggle based on differences, and instead make them "part of the global picture," as the authorized jargon has it.

A women's struggle that is not integrated into a class struggle is not valid.[64] A struggle of the disabled that does not engage the economic struggle is not recognized. It is always necessary to merge with a general consensus and rejoin the leading front of the combat. Otherwise, the word "factionalism" appears, to sanction deviant conduct.

We smile a bit now at such conceptions. But, on the one hand, this is where we are coming from, and on the other hand we cannot forget that the eclipse of analyses of the Marxist type only projected us into what is conventionally called, at the moment I write, unitarian critical thought (*la pensée unique*), and made us meekly accept a triumphant neoliberalism. Some voices were raised, denouncing the dangers of such apathy (from Cornélius Castoriadis to Michel Chauvière, including the analyses of the journal *Esprit*, etc.), but they do not make up a chorus.

"Like the others," even "like everybody else," the driving force of rehabilitation, is then the most shared, the most desired of outcomes, and bears up all the efforts directed toward disability. Some move in this direction with weak means, through compromise, creating an interplay of forces that brakes rehabilitation. Others exploit power relationships and undertake rational activism. The fact that in one or another of these forms some people can declare themselves content and furnish the conservative and paternalist conscience with good alibis, and the fact that others are completely uninterested can have nonnegligible consequences in the field and in relation to the concrete effectiveness of rehabilitation. But you will have seen that this is not my point. I say that the will to rehabilitate is a common fact on which the cultural era of the twentieth century is entirely dependent. It seems quite imprecise to be dualistic, as is a certain kind of militant thought, that is, that those who exercise public power, in particular political power, along with all the other players down to the ranks of the disabled themselves, do not have the will that I am speaking of but can only generate ideological discourse. On the other side are the objective analysts of this society, called exclusionary, who firmly hold that integration really is their aim. We must also seek out what we have at our core. I do not deny the great value of the analysis in terms of ideology. But, once we begin the search for the cultural characteristics of these epistemological divisions into historical periods, we interrogate the social oppositions themselves to determine whether a concealed will is not common to them all. Not to refuse to support either party, which is not the objective of the inquiry, but to catch the atmosphere, the hint of even more secret systems. As for the concept of will that has been used, its function is to do justice to a hidden direction and decision, of an epistemological order, recognizing a specific historical situation. When I say "of an epistemological order" I mean "which directs the manner of addressing the question in the cultural zone under consideration." The fact that the two systems, charity and liberal naturalism, can recognize both a will to integrate and the Great Effacement still says nothing about the structural organization that informs them.

This system of effacement rests, in my eyes, on the intersection of two isotopies,[65] which are substituted for two others, earlier dominant. Two levels for the reading of disability informed the arrangements and

assessments of earlier systems. The first, the biological isotopy, with
the major opposition between the normal and the abnormal (or the
monstrous). Disability was placed on the side of the abnormal, the
pathological. The normal made it possible to think of the abnormal and
then equally well made it possible to make a claim for the normative
character of the normal (the classical period). While anomaly is a
concept descriptive of variety, the normal tends toward an evaluative concept that has a referent.[66] This distinction between the normal
and the abnormal is always the product of a biological view, where
people think that they know what is natural, where the natural is
defined as *integralness, integrity.* Biologically we know what makes up
human beings: everything that they require, nothing but what they
require. But as soon as an individual has something more or something
less, he leaves biological naturalness and enters the domain of the
monstrous. The biological isotopy of which I am speaking has integrity
as its principal "seme."[67]

Added to this first register, in systems which preceded our own, is
a religious or ethical isotopy which served to axiologize, to assign
value. The abnormal and monstrous pointed to the separation between divine and evil. When this valorization was not moderated by
others, it was possible to kill the disabled, because they were abnormal, because they were bearers of misfortune. The divine/malign opposition of the religious register, intersecting that of normal/abnormal on
the biological level, provided the principle according to which certain
acts were evaluated. In a system where only the categories I have just
mentioned are in play, the physical suppression of the disabled may be
morally justified.

This religious isotopy, we have seen, was itself intersected by an
ethical isotopy, where the primary opposition was between misfortune
and good fortune. In this case, abnormality cannot be assimilated to
evil but only to misfortune. Certain systems, that of the Old Testament, for example, have shown themselves to be ethicoreligious;
others—that which prevailed in the Christian era[68]—were openly ethical. All, however, were based on a primary isotopy, the biological one.
But in the ethicoreligious case, and in opposition to the religious one
alone, nonintegralness and abnormality can no longer be suppressed;

rather, they are situated. Situated in a particular form of exclusion and integration. When we then pass to the ethical system, abnormality is not simply situated, it becomes assisted and a new form of exclusion-integration emerges.

Today, with the system of massive effacement, not only are the religious, ethicoreligious and ethical isotopies effaced, but the biological isotopy has been supplanted by a *social* isotopy. In my view, a double substitution has occurred. The biological register has become a social register, the ethicoreligious register has become a medical register. Added to this is a reversal: the medical register took up the biological register, but as an axiological register, while the social register took up the ethicoreligious register, now as the founding register. This theoretical presentation can be better understood if we approach it by setting out some concrete oppositions. As I just said, the biological level had normal and abnormal as the principal opposition. Now, the opposition that I see as fundamental is between normal and aberrant. This is a social and no longer biological opposition. For naturalness—as I have shown—is not integralness but the fact of being *integrable.* The system of the integral has given way to that of the integrable, just as the monster has yielded his place to the disabled. Even if the analysis of Georges Canguilhem remains accurate for our era, culture has already displaced the categories. In biological terms, we can, in fact, no longer very well distinguish the normal from the pathological. Blurred contours are usual. But we remain secure in the social distinction between the normalized and the marginal. The integrable and the nonintegrable are everywhere visibly marked out . . . as I have often said before. Rehabilitation medicine works more with these categories than with concepts of the normal and the pathological.

In fact, the medical isotopy is more based on the opposition between good health and poor health (or healthy/unhealthy). The concept of health is not that of normality. It is more complex on the one hand and permits an axiology on the other. We no longer speak in terms of good and evil, of divine and malign, but in terms of healthy/sickly or hygienic/harmful. There is the health promoting and the dangerous. The concept of health is medical but it also has an ethical tendency. We must seek out the healthy and get rid of what is contaminated. No one any longer uses a language of good and evil with regard to disability. But everyone uses the language of health and sickness. Medicine, which knows what health is and is there to defend it, finds itself ascribed the role that in other times fell to the cleric who knew what evil was and was charged with protecting us from it. Under the concepts of health and sickness medicine certainly still maintains the biological distinction between normal and pathological, but the drift of these concepts leads to another system. Once again, healthy/unhealthy is a less evaluative pair in social terms but much more suited to ethical judgment than the pair normal/pathological. This is why it seems to me that the system of thought presently in force can be represented in the following diagram, which shows these displacements.

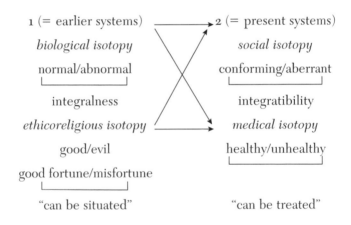

This accounts for the social division, both of the actors and of the values. In systems of the first kind, the actor is above all the priest, expert in the sacred,[69] and in certain subsystems it is legitimate to kill the disabled or give them the status of untouchables or help them. Their alterity is so reinforced and axiologized that it is recognized or expelled. In a system of the second kind—our own—the actor is doubled in the physician and the social worker (at times merged). It is no longer possible to immobilize or exterminate the disabled (but one can prevent their birth, and this is one of the directions taken by abortion as a program). They are reduced socially; they are aligned. Their difference at this point is a matter of such indifference, little axiologized on the ontological level, medicalized, that it is minimized or misrepresented. Difference could entail death or exclusion. It was overvalorized. Now difference implies disappearance and is undervalorized.

A Conclusion to Serve as Notice for the Future

Readers will have seen that my objective has been to theorize. Could the same thing have been accomplished by telling historical anecdotes? It would have been easier—and more appealing—to play up the picturesque in the creation of rehabilitation, drawing the portraits of the founders, evoking the twists and turns of their rivalries, showing how the public authorities begrudged or lavished their support. I could have brought back to life the atmosphere of Berck-Plage in the years 1925–30, with all its tubercular patients, all those "extended guests," whose horizon was the sand raised by the wind and, for many, death at the end of months of boredom. In this life at the ends of the earth some great encounters took place: Robert Buron, who became a government minister, Chapoullie who would end up a bishop, Suzanne Fouché, the founder of a great association, Louis Leprince-Ringuet who was not sick but came to give science courses. From this middle-class Catholic environment, tried by suffering and solitude, arose the will to recover and have others recover a full place in society. We could spend more time with a woman such as Madeleine Rivard, too shy and too stricken to have been able to play a public role but who was nonetheless the first person to have the great vision of reintegration into the workforce through instruction and training. She, too, founded an association that still exists. Berck gathered victims of bone tuberculosis. If the invalid did not die, her body was marked for life. It was first a question of a disease, then of a disability and continuing illness. So situated, the patients at Berck were representative of several things: they were "TB patients" and thus stricken by a disabling disease that no one knew how to cure and that had been the terror of the whole preceding century under the name of "consumption." In addition, tuberculosis was charged with symbolism, was not without dignity, and resembled in this a war wound. Tuberculosis was symbolic because it concentrated the secular ills against which society was powerless, like the plague in the fourteenth and fifteenth centuries, like syphilis in the sixteenth century, like the epidemics of the seventeenth and nineteenth centuries, and consumption and the "romantic" fevers of the nineteenth century. Symbolic also because it was dependent on the conditions of work and of life. It was like destiny, a trial, misfortune, and at the same time like poverty, vocational hazards, or collective responsibility. The tuberculosis patients who raised their voices had this symbolic capital working for them, in addition to their own energy, their religious beliefs, and membership in the bourgeoisie. Studying the Berck environment of the 1920s is to rediscover the mixed systems of which I spoke, a blend of charity, liberalism, the cult of the will, protest, and submission to the established order, but with a consciousness of being part of the national community, a bit like the disabled veterans.

But readers will also see the incompatibility of recounting a story briefly while still trying to lay out the most decisive issues. To do both would have required that I devote this entire work just to the contemporary period.

I could equally well have shown the precise genesis of rehabilitation institutions starting with the war of 1914. It is stimulating to consider the birth of the huge village of Clairvivre in Dordogne. The idiosyncratic and stubborn Albert Delsuc wanted to make Clairvivre into a kind of health commune, where the tubercular patients, in exchange for work, would receive vouchers in order to procure what they wanted from a general store. The project did not quite develop in that sense but Clairvivre did become a community of the disabled and continues to this day. Delsuc had a talent for drawing enormous sums of money from the authorities in order to make Clairvivre a place and a time of transition between the sanatorium and normal life, through the process of rehabilitation for work. This project had been made possible by the creation of schools during the war years under the auspices of the national office for disabled veterans. They had more than two thousand trainees undergoing therapy in 1932. This means that in the context of veterans and various other victims of war (widows as well as the injured) therapy and rehabilitation were immediately matters of general and basic consensus, even if legislation on behalf of all the disabled had to wait, and central administrations were slow and rigid.

In this summary account of the large associations that were founded in this rush of activity, I should mention the birth of Auxilia (1925), Ladapt (1929), the Association of Paralytics of France (1934). The last-named is today one of the most powerful and its founder, André Trannoy (a quadriplegic), like the founder of Ladapt, Suzanne Fouché (bone tuberculosis and burns), died only recently. Along with others, they struggled to create facilities of different kinds (schools, physical therapy centers, vocational centers, sheltered workshops, social services, etc.). After 1945 centers run by health insurance unions would be grafted on to all these arrangements that only continued to expand.

Parallel to all this we should give an account of the history of institutions for developmentally retarded children or adults: the Croix Marines in 1935, the Adapei (regional associations of the parents of disabled children), later united in a powerful national association (Unapei, created in 1960). The sector of maladjusted youth was added during the war years of 1939 to 1945. It was oriented toward social cases just as well as toward disability and developmental retardation. To all of this which I have evoked so summarily I should add many *et ceteras* so that none of the great initiators feels forgotten. But such an enumeration becomes taxing. From all these allusions I isolate the fact that after a starting point that was almost public, the vast majority of institutions are now in private hands, although under the guardianship and control of various ministries (Health, Labor, and today National Solidarity or Vocational Training). This private character also returns us to the double system of charity (secularized) and liberalism (accommodated).

But readers should be warned: they would have been able to follow the course of such a history more easily, but it would have been infinitely more difficult to understand what has underpinned rehabilitation for the last sixty years. The deep-seated will, proclaimed and concealed at the same time, to reintegrate as much as possible and thus to make disability into something banal, with all its variety mixed together, is not conveyed by a simple account.

The networks that make up the system of relationships between present-day society and anomaly can be exposed only by linking up the day-to-day practices, legislation, the ways of identifying and designating disability, the administrative arrangements. On this basis, then, we have a duty to elaborate, conceptualize, theorize. Despite the rather numerous historical indications to the contrary, working all this out seems to presuppose that the factual history of events is already well-known. Public opinion today is generally rather well informed about the large-scale legal arrangements, types of institutions, and principal administrative structures. If this were not the case—and many specialists think that it is not despite efforts by the media—I would say that the detailed account of past decades would not provide much material relevant to the problem that I wished to raise.

This problem has a number of aspects. First, how is one to classify and divide the disabled? Certainly the major distinctions—sensory, motor, mental (in several senses), social—remain useful. But I have wished to focus on the tendency toward fusion into a generic "disabled person." Similarly, through this process of lexical impoverishment, categories which particularly in antiquity had nothing to do with one another—congenital, adventitious—have been brought together. It is certainly the case that on the level of individual psychology the difference between disability from birth and an accident in the course of life is very strongly felt. But on the level of social treatment this difference is erased, and we find everyone in the same organizations, subject to the same rules, claiming the same rights. The distinction between mental, psychological, and physical itself tends to be erased. Not initially because one can be associated with another by all kinds of processes and for all sorts of reasons (in particular, psychological disorders and physical disability), but principally because the same regulations, the same social expectations, the same kinds of assistance are directed toward them all. Obviously, we must note that psychiatric illness and mental retardation have not experienced the same fate in the recent past. Mental illness is treated in psychiatric hospitals and within its own sector. Mental disability in the narrow sense, such as low intelligence quotient, Down's syndrome, etc., is not treated within the confines of the psychiatric hospital, but in specialized institutions. These facilities—like those for the disabled— vary: group homes, centers for assistance through employment, medical-educational institutes or medical-vocational institutes for youth, etc. Often the foundations or associations are specialized in terms of the kind of mental disorder.

But all these distinctions have in no way prevented a psychiatrization of these establishments, unless they are just pure and simple improvements on the hospice, that is, hostels with some few activities. Psychiatrists and special education experts share the tasks, roles, and power. Everywhere we see the movement to which I have been calling attention: rehabilitation. In extreme cases where it is only a matter of providing shelter this is little felt, by the very nature of the institution, but the fact remains that as soon as a chance opens up, some agency attempts educational, social, and vocational reinsertion.

In this overall picture, we must be sure not to forget all the experience that could be grouped under the heading antipsychiatry. The simplest and neatest definition of antipsychiatry was given by D. Cooper when he spoke of "being oneself with others." The objective here, under formulas of different kinds, is to return the aberrant to social life but by making the social group accept the aberration in question. Antipsychiatry is presented as an effort to forge an integration without erasing difference, without wanting to efface or reduce the "abnormality." Of course, by this brokered contact between the aberrant and the social group, antipsychiatry sees itself as therapeutic: the psychiatrist is not absent from antipsychiatry, ill-named as it is. But in the great proponents such as Cooper, Laing, Mannoni, we can distinguish much more than an ambition to cure or adapt. For them it is a matter of reconstituting *sociability,* that is, living together in difference. The antipsychiatric project, in its impetus, is a project to reconstitute the social fabric, to give life back to concrete relationships of difference, while the whole movement of industrial society, the nuclear family, individual housing, breaks down basic sociability, dichotomizes the population. In effect, in order to live in the family as it is conceived, in housing as it is manufactured, in the business world as it gives rhythm to time and space, people are obliged to separate themselves from the elderly, and at times from the young, to consign their children in difficulty to specialists, to exclude from their homes the retarded or disabled. All weaknesses, aberrations, maladjustments are revealed as incompatible with the organization of daily life, in particular in its urban form. And so retirement homes flourish, gilded cages to confine the old folks; institutions for the mentally retarded, group homes for those with mental disorders; establishments for the disabled, concentrations of "not like the rest"; and so on for every category that is no longer in the mainstream, that is prevented from living under conditions that have been created for the average and for the majority.

Antipsychiatry has seen all this. Antipsychiatry also wants integration, but by economizing—to the maximum—on what I have called therapy and rehabilitation. That is, it does not want to take the aberrant person in order to render her apt to rejoin the crowd called normal, but it tries to graft the branch that was rejected because of maladjustment back onto the ordinary trunk, requiring from the latter an adaptation to difference. This shading of viewpoint is actually a gulf of difference! Is this a dream? Like every bold—and optimistic—thought, it will have to make its way through difficult and unforeseen ins and outs. Is it perhaps just a dream to interpret antipsychiatry in this sense?

In addition, I think I perceive something similar in the protests coming from minority groups of the disabled. In a general way, the disabled are relatively passive before the institutions that I have outlined. Some seek as well as they can individual solutions to the issue of compensation.[70] Politicized protest groups have been formed,[71] and they radically challenge the whole complex of legislation and institutions. Through political and social analyses, whose schematic nature must be recognized, I believe that I can make out the underlying protest: "we are not asking for our difference to be forgotten, because we are 'disabled' and we know it, but we challenge integration, rehabilitation that works by labeling, specialized treatment, aid—all intended to make producing-consuming agents of us." Put another way, we want *our place*, and not a place that has been designated for us, similar and different, equal and different, disabled but able (valid, valorized, validated). It is not a simple matter to find a common language with these groups because violence—the violence of mimesis, as Girard would say—is so great. Impatience has been aggravated. But in my analysis, these are heralds of a new historical change. This is equally the meaning that must be ascribed to the powerful movements today in Italy, Quebec, and Denmark, which insist on deinstitutionalization and devocationalization—barbarous words to indicate that this is the end of normative adjustment and the cycle that I have called effacement by means of specialization alone. Will this dawn turn into a real day? What will be the system that establishes itself? Analysis is not prophecy.

Fifteen years after these concluding lines, which I have not changed, must I disavow them and admit that all that has been forgotten? I insisted at the time on new movements directly intended for adults and on integration in employment. The history of agencies devoted to children, the question of school integration, polarization on the issue of the eradication of genetic disease, are still to be evoked. The model of rehabilitation and of disability to which I devoted my effort is now perhaps in retreat, confronted with the questions posed by multiple disability, diseases of the genome, AIDS. Similarly, antipsychiatry, as such, has retired in the same way as analyses like Foucault's. But at the same time, on the social side a new notion of exclusion has returned to force, in the form of the double event of unemployment and of changes in sexual and family habits. But for all that, the force of what came into play as a consequence of work accidents, war injuries, the generalization of social security, on the one hand, and movements challenging classical psychiatry (even if the latter was saved by medication), challenging a society that is selective, reproductive, normalizing, directive, on the other hand—none of all this can be whisked away, as if we were starting again at zero. It is the historian's role to prevent the social group from falling into amnesia, as it is to denounce what is modish, simple cosmetic change, significant losses of memory. There certainly exist deep divides that may be operative under our eyes without our seeing them, but the precondition for seeing them is to know well what has gone before. It is for this reason that I have retained these pages that I wrote fifteen years ago.

Epilogue

Should I deny myself the right to make proposals? Let us admit that the foregoing analysis—like all analyses—hardly prepares me to do so. It does not prepare me because it reveals the weight of systems of thoughts and of complexes of mental attitudes. The historical variations are considerable, and my effort has been expended on the moments of rupture. But readers will have noted how these divides are not self-determined: they occur under the pressure of new discourses and new historical circumstances (material, ideal, or imaginary). It is not even sure that it is possible to account for them. They are observed. Explanations are always weak, even when given in the belief that it is "social science" that is being done, as certain Marxist thought believes. We are, rather, confronted by a moving mass whose displacement factors are unknown to us. From this we can gain an idea of the historical structures but must renounce any ambition toward universal comprehension or a permanent perspective.

How, under these circumstances, can we think that suggestions for action and organization can have any effect? Systems of thought and the directions taken by social practice are so little dependent on us!

Yet there is another aspect that my analysis has revealed. This is the importance of discourse, of language, of texts. Without oversubscribing to notions of the will, it is possible to risk believing that saying is also doing. I have already stated what I thought of the relationship between discourse and praxis: not a relationship in which the one reflects or expresses the other but a kind of interweave. Social praxis also consists of generating discourse, which is not at all to say that there is no distinction.

My discourse, readers will have understood, will be that of difference. Constantly facing this phenomenon, societies have never succeeded in integrating difference *as such.* Either the social group integrates difference in order to make it disappear or integrates partially while excluding certain forms even more, or it excludes radically while paying lip service to a conception of integration. We cannot take any one of the formulas that history has chosen at a given moment and erect it into an ideal. Each path, in its own context, has had its advantages and has known limitations. Today the will to assimilate, to trivialize by an intense circumscription and treatment, cannot be challenged. But, in addition, I can see in these intentions the risk of make-believe, of doing "as if," despite the outlay of impressive financial and technological support. It thus seems to me that we must attempt to think an integration *out from* difference.

Perhaps you could try to convince me that on the practical level this is already in progress. The preceding analysis proves that this is not at all the case. We are bringing difference back to the norm. Or, at least, we are trying to do so. In more theoretical terms some people would say that the problem itself is poorly conceived. We could, in fact, argue about the concept of difference. After all, we have such a concept in our minds for the simple reason that we have an idea of a norm and of normality. A difference is designated as such only in relation to something from which it differs. This is why I must generalize the concept: there are only differences, as Saussure said of language. Everything is different from everything else. Put another way, we are in a world of singularities. Thus, there are no longer the able and the disabled, just as there is no longer any reason distinct from unreason, imaginary distinct from ideal, body separated from spirit, practice separated from discourse. Society is made up only of "relatives" and relationships. But grasping this, still on the theoretical level, scarcely gets us anywhere. Suppressing the fixed points is possible only in total abstraction, since, in fact, historically, there are always dividing lines, as arbitrary and culturally determined as you like but no less inevitable and necessary. On the other hand, stating that there is nothing but singularities that are relative to one another presents problems of every order. Isn't this the same thing as creating a new universal, albeit a vague one? Isn't this breaking society into tiny pieces and making it unmanageable? Isn't it—the supreme paradox—fixing differences and particularities as atoms, monads, absolutes?

I cannot reply here in detail to these objections. I would only say that we can sustain the thought of difference by basing it in the radical nature of the idea itself. That is, difference is never fixed because it is a relationship. No doubt the relation of "something" to "something else," but this something was itself constituted by the relationship and is always in a state of instability dependent on the network in which it is implicated.

Let us take an example, perhaps the most difficult one. Man and woman differ, and many have wished and still wish today that they could live without dominating each other, without assimilating, but also without forming two fixed states, two new natures. Two objections can be raised immediately. Their differences, no matter how evident, rest on a profound identity: both are human, with the same intellectual, moral, psychological capacity, etc. The difference is secondary in relation to their common membership in the human species. This is equality in one respect, because they are fundamentally identical! The difference between the sexes is, after all, only a kind of accident that must doubtless be managed but which cannot be allowed to structure the relationship as a whole. For the moment I shall pass over the social consequences that could be drawn from this vision, since the accidental can permit a dichotomy between a theoretical recognition, common to us all, and the practice of exploitation. Second objection: if we emphasize the difference, breaking the unity of the human, we make sexual difference the fundamental one and make the two protagonists into two natures. This is still equality, perhaps, but a very abstract one, since they are not similar and have no need to seek to resemble each other nor to acquire what the other possesses, makes, or creates.

We must admit that the problem is not well focused. Biology and anatomy, no more than sociological habits or ancestral divisions, ought not to serve as fixed reference points. Nor should we conceive of a humanity that transcends the two sexes. The biological data, point of departure both for the common species and the difference between the sexes—to use a very old terminology—are to be conceived of in their respective spheres of influence and in the networks in which they are located. Sex is only a progressive differentiation. The anatomical and biological result of feminine and masculine characteristics is not a great matter in itself without the face-to-face relationship, the psychological and sociological interplay that begins even before birth. In all of this there is neither identity nor separation. If we are aware of the processes, of all kinds, that make us man or woman, we will never understand the idea of a unique nature nor that of two natures. We will understand only a "virilization" and "feminization," thus, a singularization and individuation—with, at times, all the well-known ambiguities and ambivalences on one level or another. Thinking the man-woman difference correctly seems to constrain thinking relationship, process, singularity, individuality: all this *together* and *on different levels.* We think process, and so evolution, and so historicity, and so the possibility of something new, but never starting from nothing. We always already have a past, a history, a sociohistorical given. If not predetermined, we are not without preconditions.

Let us stop seeing the able and disabled as normality and aberration, and let us no longer set them out as two separate kinds. What will *our* discourse be? Let us try to envisage a new historical variation from this position.

We will not demand of the disabled person that she resemble an able person. We will not make a person who is disabled into someone inherently disabled, more or less below the normal. Like the male/female face-to-face, the relationship between sound and less sound will always be treated relatively, dynamically, differently. This is the direction of future thought. On the level of action this perspective should have important consequences.

What would be the steering principles of financing? What would be desirable types of organizational structures and institutions? What are to be the forms of the relationship between the state and actions directed toward the disabled?

It seems to me that the premise we ought to establish, in order both to avoid exclusion and to recognize difference, should be: never to uproot, remove, withdraw, a child or adult struck by destiny from her or his original, living environment.[1]

I insist on this premise before responding to some very real difficulties. The best integration will always be the first one and not reintegration after a long, specialized movement through the circuit. If we want to integrate, let's not disintegrate in order to reintegrate!

At the same time, acceptance of and the greatest respect for difference are not to be expected from collective social structures but from immediate social surroundings. There is everything to be won by directing maximum effort toward the specific point of origin, most often the home, so that it may retain subjects afflicted with malformation, disabling illness, other impairments.

To judge by the evidence, this is difficult and for three principal reasons. The first reason is far-reaching: contemporary society disaggregates sociability. The nuclear family requires living in limited space, preferably urban. Employment and training call for preparations, conversions, modifications, that entail adjustments in both time and space. Leisure activities, access to supplies and culture, etc., that presuppose mobility, schedules, flexibility, which are often incompatible with the awkwardness, physical and mental weakness. The list could be made longer.

The second reason that this uprooting seems required is the technological constraints of the care, medical follow-up, therapy sessions of all kinds, surgical intervention, etc. How, for example, can you keep at home a myopathic child who, if he is to live and have a long life, must do directed daily exercises for walking, breathing, posture, who must from time to time undergo surgery requiring preliminary observation, the operation itself, convalescence? In short, large-scale medical and educational techniques come at high cost and often require being torn away from the ordinary environment of life.

There is a third reason for expelling the aberrant from the basic group: the psychological difficulty of tolerating the affected person. This third reason is to be closely associated with the first, because the psychological tolerance of a community depends to a great extent on its vitality and sociological viability. It is evident, for example, that if the mother alone must bear almost all the constraints while the husband is outside the home (work, errands, participation in civic life, etc.), if other children claim their own legitimate rights, if the environment is made up only of distant and pitying greetings—"hello, how are we today?"—the situation is intolerable. My example is only an example; there are a thousand other circumstances that, by their non-sociability, make the obstacles to having a disabled person at home insurmountable. Beyond these sociological factors, however, we must recognize the internal difficulty of living continuously with an impaired person.

Finally, we can advance a fourth reason: it is often necessary, for one's psychological health, to leave one's original environment in order to gain personal autonomy. In such a case passage through an institution, at least temporarily, is of great value.

So, what has happened to my hypothesis of leaving the disabled in their vital home environment? This remains for me the *objective*, on the condition that we implement a series of actions to make this possible on a regular basis. For there will always be moments when one must have recourse to a specialized process.

All these actions could tend in the direction of personalized assistance, as close as possible to these base environments. To provide space—and accessible space—to a family that has a wheelchair; subsidize the material and educational arrangements for schools on the level of local governmental units (according to the geography), so that, except in exceptional cases or during short-term hospital stays, disabled children are *integrally* among others; in parallel, to have frameworks for physical therapy or psychological aid well distributed in geographical terms, adjoining school facilities for example. This same principle would be valid for vocational training on the secondary educational level. And, in principle, having centers for the vocational training of adults opened to the disabled presents no problems providing that there is a firm political will (and strict control) always to take difference into account. This presupposes some work of conversion within institutions now as oriented toward uniformity as the Department of National Education or the Association for the Vocational Training of Adults.[2]

It is evident that the logic outlined here entails many specialized institutions.3 We must be lucid and respond that many of the present workers in these institutions could do similar work in other settings. But these institutions also require reassurance, for, in the range of actions that have to be undertaken close to the disabled persons and their home group, they will still have a great deal to do but in a new spirit and subsequent to conversions of various kinds. It is very evident that if these private sector associations were really federated, coordinated, and steered in a common direction and toward flexibility, everyone would stand to win. One of the missions of these service providers would be, in fact, to convince people that the most humane course of action is to live with those who are different from the majority and to facilitate all the small ways to make this concretely possible.

There remains, in addition, the need for some large-scale medical and surgical framework for operations and treatments dependent on advanced technology. Equally unavoidable are certain institutions for cases with no real solution in physical, psychological, or mental terms. Admission to such facilities should be a rigorously administered process, and substantial resources should be available so that the disabled can later leave them with a view to resuming group social life in their original surroundings. Such structures, instead of becoming commonplace, should remain exceptional.

It is also within the framework of integration in the home environment that work placement policies should be developed, with a recognized priority accorded to such integration, even if it means being less obsessed with salaried work of the industrial kind. In addition, a program of aid to businesses could have as its objective to get impaired persons working as such, without putting them on equal footing with others, without penalizing them, without obliging them to the same demands as others. A number of work formulas could be devised. This presupposes the necessary budget allocations, well-studied financial aid systems that are adaptable to concrete cases. The funding is above all a question of judicious distribution.

When setting out these grand, general objectives, I have no doubt that I run the risk of appearing a soft-headed utopian or a hard-hearted spoiler. You could just as well make fun of someone who is sawing off the branch he is sitting on, since the author himself has lived in the framework of specialized institutions. *Tout beau!* Steady now! as they would have said in the century of Louis XIV. I am pointing out a horizon, without casting recriminations, without claiming that I can act directly in conformity with my own personal thoughts. Moreover, the orientation that I propose is simple: set in motion processes and initiatives so that the social fabric is amenable to accepting difference. In order to do this, we have to check the movement that animates all our Western society: setting aside in order to make disappear, and reintegrating, often artificially and by requiring a nonerasable effacement. Some people in some parts of the world have understood this, and actions of this kind have been undertaken in Italy, in Quebec, and at times in France.

Nor should this orientation appear as a complete program. Mediation is difficult, never completely satisfactory, always slow. It would be too easy to pull things down, to create scapegoats (associations, authorities, the disabled, physicians, families . . .). Thus, my last suggestion would be for an advocacy movement concerned with informing public opinion and with drafting proposals. It would be made up of the people whose bodies and minds are affected and would be broadly supported by public agencies that would agree to fund a Great Laboratory charged with taking up questions in their most fundamental form. Our societies have invented the principle of social security; they have recognized trade unionism; they have discovered rewarding formulas for the coordination of efforts. Why could they not invent a new way to nurture difference, with a clear view of its essence and its appearance, without subjecting it, without giving up?

I have intentionally limited myself to a few generalities. It would be vain, at the end of a book like this, to announce and advance a series of concrete reforms. But I want to put the objectives that I have submitted as *radical* requests into a larger perspective.

I have spoken of "sociability" (*sociabilité*), which others call "sociality" (*socialité*). The acceptance of a person afflicted, whether congenitally or otherwise, whether physically or mentally, presupposes work on the life environment and thus a search for sociability. We are caught, in most of our societies (less so in the Scandinavian social democracies), between a state with a providential character and a privatization of the refuge kind. The stronger individualistic privatization, the greater the demand on the state to provide services and funding. The more the state extends its sway, the more room the private takes up in defense. I subscribe to the thinking of those who believe that we can effect a "rapprochement of society with itself."[4] Not through the dream of a kind of community-based counter-society but by promoting innumerable local collective solidarities, on issues ranging from taxation to social justice, passing through all kinds of services, yet not bureaucratized nor centralized. Obviously, I cannot develop this social thinking here. It may also find support in the capacity for resistance of numerous social groups that face the aggression of the state or of individualism. As Agnès Pitrou has shown, there are, for example, underground networks of family solidarity; in periods of crisis hidden economies, "black markets," develop. Under certain conditions social spaces, public without being statist, differential without being individualistic, may arise or be created, and there is a fertile ground, thus far scarcely noticed, for this to happen.

It is in such a framework, only the salient features of which I have noted, that societal action on behalf of the disabled would be situated. I do not believe that creating communities of the disabled, even with a humanist and spiritual foundation, is a solution that is possible on a large scale. Certainly, we can only admire the work of a Jean Vanier, but I do not believe in the societal mission of such formulas as his. The antipsychiatric community, provided that it does not become locked into inward-looking, community-based stances and retains its mediating function, can easily be in the vanguard. Nor is it membership in the base communities of the able that I would advocate, even though they are quite capable of integrating this or that disabled person while respecting difference. The effort and direction that seem most promising to me are a reduction in demands on the state, as P. Ronsavallon says, and a multiplication of "on-the-spot public services based on local initiative." There is not, we must admit, any pure model of this third way; only a complex overlapping is feasible. I simply wanted to situate the frame of reference where I would locate myself. Moreover, we should note that past initiatives (such as the Adapei for mentally

impaired children) fit quite well into such a perspective. But institutionalization has ended up by consuming its original goals because of
the requirements of administration and organization. This has a great
deal to do with its private association character, which has had to face
financial and corporatist challenges. It would then be a question, in
the perspective that I have outlined, of letting the state play a role in
activating various forms of solidarity but as a support for a basic solidarity, expanded through series of deconcentrated subsystems and "directly borne by concrete social relationships" (Rosanvallon). Neither
locked in specialized circuits nor refugees in warm-hearted communities nor left to individualist aid, disabled people would belong to
organizations that had been socialized in the fabric of the short-range
actions that shape society at its fundamental stage. Today, rereading
my earlier conclusion, I persist in holding these views in the full
knowledge that an evolution, perhaps a real breakthrough, has occurred, is in the process of occurring. The end of a book sets a new
date for the future.

Appendix: Stages in the Legislation

Let us recall here some of the legislative history as concerns our central topic of rehabilitation, with no claim to exhaustiveness, since the body of regulations is so ample.

This will set out only the main lines, or, rather, the main periods. The era before World War I was described earlier. A first period, roughly the years 1920–30, establishes the principal concepts: January 2, 1918, the law concerning vocational therapy and the national office of the war wounded and medically discharged; March 1919 and April 1924, a general law on assistance for vocational redeployment, complemented by the law of May 5, 1924, authorizing the admission of those with work-related injuries to the schools of therapy for the war wounded. An analogous extension on May 14, 1930.

The second period, however curious this may first seem, runs until 1957. Policy was directed at creating structures that would correspond to the first idea of rehabilitation and to concepts that had appeared at the end of the war. We should point out the merging of these notions with those prevalent in neighboring sectors, such as that of children: in 1935 governmental decrees concerning wards of the court gave priority to rehabilitative placement and coordinated a whole series of initiatives, both preventive and integrating, that had been taken at this time in the area of children at risk (for this period and for World War II, see M. Chauvière, *Enfance inadaptée, l'héritage de Vichy* [Éd. de l'Atélier / Éd. Ouvrières, 1980]). The period of German occupation under the Vichy government, even if it played only a minor role for the physically impaired (only a single decree can be noted, from July 1, 1942, dealing with the aptitude of candidates for training), in practice created the concept of "maladjusted children." This discovery would join other maladjustments and contribute to broaden the concept of disability to all areas.

On July 27, 1942, a law on children's courts and observation centers sought to create a private arrangement for the management of the delinquent population with reception centers, observations centers, rehabilitation centers, although a very rigorous correctional framework was maintained in the public sector. This was the intention of the children's protection and rescue plan of November 1941, due to the abbé Jean Plaquevent. Even though this continued to be a segregating practice by virtue of its screening, M. Chauvière writes: "Here humanitarian needs have been overrun in the interests of a practice that made a comprehensive appeal to *technicity* and whose only justification would be in technicity itself. From a generous guardianship there slowly emerges a rationalization for the cost coverage system" (53). Created on July 25, 1943, was the Technical Council for Delinquent, Morally Threatened Youth, which would establish the primacy of child neuropsychiatry in the field of delinquent youth but would adopt the notion of *maladjusted children*, ready for readjustment. A public debate on social and vocational reentry was begun, tied to the eugenics program and work ideology of the Vichy government. Whatever credit may be given to this debate and its political undertones, and the scant effect exercised by the economic necessity of reintroducing maladjusted youth to employment, these ideas, spread during the occupation years, would come to haunt the entire postwar period. But their origins lie earlier: they were taken over and applied to a domain scarcely relevant to them until then. Schools of rehabilitators saw the light of day during the occupation, linked with the creation of Arsea (regional associations for the safety of children and adolescents). The discourse was certainly corporatist and depoliticized, and the working class did not join it. It was a mixture of technicity, statism, fascism, family values, in short, a moral/technical synthesis. Nonetheless, the tradition of private works of charitable assistance was shattered in quite radical fashion. In the postwar period, and to return to the disabled themselves, we must underline the importance of governmental decrees from 1945 affecting social security and a regulation from October 31 of the same year concerning the vocational redeployment of people with tuberculosis. One year later (October 30, 1946) a law provided for the vocational rehabilitation of victims of work-related accidents. In 1949 the Cordonnier law was passed (August 2). The concept of rehabilitation finally took effective form, in a context where union and political militants played a very important role, in particular through the administration of the social security offices, where they had the dominant place. Rehabilitation, at one stroke, is removed both from the encapsulation of the simple charitable perspective of the church-run establishments and from the grip of governmental control with its totalitarian or exclusively technical tendency. Claims for the rights of disabled persons will henceforth take the upper hand. But the fundamental plan had not varied since its first appearance: reintegration.

The decades of the 1950s and 1960s are peppered with texts that I shall not list in detail, intended either to create certain types of structures and institutions or to widen the possibilities for impaired persons (especially in financial terms) or else to put business under the obligation to provide employment.

A third period is inaugurated by the law of November 23, 1957, an organically conceived law that systematized the right to work, provided a definition of the disabled worker, created a high council for social and vocational redeployment, and imposed a new disabled employment quota on businesses. From this moment on, the legislative labyrinth grows to such an extent that we would get lost in the details. Here I would refer to some of the more accessible accounts: A. Labregère, *Les Personnes handicapées. Notes et études documentaires* (1976); or a document from the Ministry of Labor, *La Législation française et les handicapés;* or S. Fouché, *Les Étapes d'une législation* (Cahiers de Ladapt 1973), 44. We should also note the importance of a report prepared by F. Bloch-Lainé in 1967.

I have investigated the intersection of the fields of maladjustment and disability. The rather purist formulation that prevailed for several decades of how maladjustment was to be figured is found in *Nomenclature et classification des jeunes inadaptés* (Nomenclature and Classification of Maladjusted Youth), which appeared in *Sauvegarde,* nos. 2–4, in 1946, from the pens of the high priests of French psychology and pedagogy of the time: Lagache, Dechaume, Dublineau, Girard, Guillemain, Heuyer, Launay, Male, Préaut, Wallon. "Maladjusted refers to a child, adolescent, or more generally a young adult of less than 21 years of age, whose lack of aptitude or defects of character put into prolonged conflict with reality and the requirements of his or her surroundings relative to the age and social environment of the young person." One could hardly more clearly attribute maladjustment to the almost natural characteristics of the individual, who is obliged to realign herself with the norms of her reference group, without the latter being in the least interrogated as to the maladjustment. The field of disability will then come into conflict with this definition to the extent that it will increasingly be defined as the social consequence of a deficiency or incapacity, otherwise unpredictable and accidental.

The principal service rendered by Bloch-Lainé's report from 1968, *De l'inadaptation des personnes handicapées* (On the Maladjustment of the Disabled) was to distinguish the factors that stem from the environment and to make specific the association of disability with deficiency. This report was the cornerstone for the discussions that preceded the passage of the law of 1975. The study completed by Bloch-Lainé is paralleled by that begun at the same time by Philip Wood, as commissioned by the World Health Organization, which led in 1980 to the adoption of the *Classification internationale des handicaps: déficience, incapacité, désavantage, un manuel de classification des conséquences des maladies* (CTNRHL-Inserm, 1988). A great deal of ink has flowed over this study, which has become a kind of bible and has influenced concrete measures that have been taken. The major distinctions are henceforth known. I shall limit myself to a few remarks. However useful, even necessary, the distinctions set out in this document are not completely original: it is a codification of what the very word *handicap* had introduced and what common sense could work out. This classificatory document betrays its medical origins, and the efforts, furthered polemically by Quebeckers, to have the level of disadvantage, or "handicap," developed and assume more importance and autonomy, are to be encouraged. The relatively pragmatic character of the classification conceals a deeper analysis, in sociological or anthropological terms, of the collective figuring of disability and of what the issues are in this domain. To take this study as the ultimate theoretical elaboration would be to camouflage many aspects of the field as seen by Bourdieu, that is, as a domain of conflict over rights and powers, over privilege and status, etc. This classification has at times generated real intellectual laziness. Finally, we should not forget the difference between the original English title and the French translation, which was not ready to abandon the use of the word *handicap* as a generic term, while the English simply says *International Classification of Impairments, Disabilities and Handicaps*.

To this third period I would readily assign the characteristic feature of having broadened—or given—the means to the final reintegration, after the second period had put in place the structure to permit rehabilitation. In any case there is a great deal of arbitrariness in any periodization, as long as one is not working on a true epistemological level. Let us accept periods as a convenience, nothing more.

A fourth period can be identified starting with the law of July 13, 1971. This is the period of benefits! This law established new benefits: benefits to disabled adults and benefits to disabled minors, followed by a housing allowance. Jumping over numerous governmental decrees and circulars that sought to effect integration in social life or salaried employment, I must mention the law of 1975, which made three major kinds of dispositions: revamped benefits, new administrative structures, modified arrangements for salaried employment. There was a plethora of interpretations and critiques of this law. Among others, readers may refer to the report on the legislation in *Droits des personnes handicapées*, ed. P. Verdier (ESF Éditeur, 1979). For a critical analysis the unpublished report edited by Bloch-Lainé is severe but is not in fundamental disagreement. (The same applies to the report of the Economic and Social Council.)

These two official reports should not make us forget the report from the early 1980s issued by a subcommittee on rationalization of budget options (RCB). Presenting itself as imaginative (many suggestions are made) and not lacking in an attractive generosity (train and place a greater number of disabled workers), it takes the very type of stance that I call "appearances only": extend services to the disabled, but by specifying them less and less and by trying to make disability *negligible* for society, that is, to deny and negate it. On this, see Michel Chauvière and Alain Durand-Davian, "Entre humanisme et technocratie," *Informations Sociales* (1979): 415.

Since the beginning of the 1980s many reports have been commissioned by the relevant administrations—more to evaluate the arrangements that derived from the law of 1975 than the law itself, as is logical for administrations. All parties accommodated themselves to the law, trying to make the best of it. The analysis that I offer need not limit itself in the same fashion. As concerns integration into an ordinary environment, its impact has been sufficiently weak that it provoked a reactivation of the legislation from 1957 on corporate obligations to provide employment for the disabled (the law of July 10, 1987). This stimulated many reports in its turn. An analysis of the hesitations, ambivalences, and ambiguities of the entire operation to reintroduce the disabled to employment is found in Alain Blanc, *Les Handicapés au travail, analyse sociologique d'un dispositif d'insertion professionelle* (Dunod, 1995).

Notes

Chapter 1

1. I am alluding to the "new philosophers," as they are called, who, like B.-H. Levy in *Le Testament de Dieu*, claim that beyond Jewish monotheism there is only barbarity.

2. See, for example, the moving testimony of Francine Fredet under the title *Mais Madame, vous êtes la mère* . . . (Le Centurion, 1979).

3. Consider, for example, the machinery of the regional "departmental commissions," responsible for counseling the disabled (CDES, Cotorep, etc.).

4. Genesis, principally chapter 1. But chapter 2 (the second account of creation) is no less significative; see P. Beauchamp, *Création et séparation* (Éditeurs Groupés, 1970).

5. I borrow this phrasing from Clément Rosset, in a short philosophical essay, *L'Objet singulier* (Éditions de Minuit, 1979), 41.

6. Georges Canguilhem, "La Monstruosité et le monstrueux." *Diogène* 40, no. 29 (1962).

7. "It is monstrosity and not death that is the vital countervalue. Death is the permanent, unconditional menace of decomposition of the organism, it is limitation from without, the negation of the living by the non-living. But monstrosity is the accidental and conditional menace of incompleteness or of distortion in shaping the form, it is limitation from within, the negation of the living by the nonviable" (Canguilhem, "La Monstruosité et le monstrueux," 31).

8. Clinical experimentation, in step with theory, and reinforced by studies related to social figurations, tells us that this is so. The major works, found in the appended bibliography, are the studies of Sausse, Assouly-Piquet, Giami, Oé, and Paicheler.

9. It would be necessary to distinguish the problematics of difference from those of alterity. See Jean Baudrillard, *La Transparence du mal, essai*

sur les phénomènes extrêmes (Galilée, 1990). On the historical level the break is apparent between the era before the French Revolution, when the problematics of alterity permitted the practice of reclusion and tolerance at the same time, and the process of democratization, in the register of difference and inclusion, but with the enormous difficulty of making such separation viable in one and the same public space. How can someone who is politically autonomous be internally alienated? On this question, see the work of Marcel Gauchet and Gladys Swain, in particular *Dialoguer avec l'insensé* (Gallimard, 1994).

10. Here I employ, in summary form, the works of René Girard, *La Violence et le sacré* (Grasset, 1972) and *Des choses cachées depuis la fondation du monde* (Fasquelle, 1978).

11. As witness, I would cite Claude Veil, *Handicap et société* (Flammarion, 1968). Two pages are devoted to the history of the word and to the field of *handicap* and not a single history book is cited in the bibliography. This was not the aim of the book, but it does show how little historical inquiry was being conducted at the time. Things have certainly changed in the last thirty years. It is beyond the scope of a note to review the relevant literature. In my doctoral thesis (unpublished) I attempted to lay out a course for future research, and the notes that follow bear witness to this. I would cite two publications as landmarks: "De l'infirmité au handicap, jalons historiques," *Cahiers du CTNERHI* 50 (April–June 1990); and H.-J. Stiker, M. Vial, and C. Barral, eds., *Handicap et inadaptation, fragments pour une histoire, notions et acteurs* (Alter, 1996). Such studies show that historical research is making progress, however slowly.

12. Guy-H. Allard, ed., *Aspects de la marginalité au Moyen Âge* (Éditions de l'Aurore, 1975).

13. The typology of science that I summarize here is drawn from this author. G. G. Grangier's opus is vast. My inspiration is Grangier, "Événement et structure dans les sciences de l'homme," *Cahiers de l'Institut des Sciences Économiques Appliquées* 55 (1957).

14. Paul Veyne, *Comment on écrit l'histoire, suivi de Foucault révolutionne l'histoire* (Le Seuil, 1978).

15. René-Claude Lachal, "Infirmes et infirmités dans les proverbes italiens," *Ethnologie Française* 2, nos. 1–2 (1972). As before, this would have to be extended by a relatively long bibliographical review; see the titles cited at the end of this work. In terms of the history of anthropology, relevant elements may be found in the studies of Jacquelin Gateaux-Mennecier, André Michelet, Gary Woodill, Philippe Caspar, Harlan Lane, Jacques Postel and Claude Quétel, and Claude Wacjman. We should never forget the fundamental book of Erving Goffman. More recent are: J.-S. Morvan and H. Paicheler, *Représentations et handicaps,*

and the special issue of *Sciences sociales et santé* 12, no 1 (March 1994). Recent studies that have been completed are by Giami, Denise Jodelet, P. Boiral, J.-P. Brouat, Gardou, Saladin, Casanova, and Vidali. To these should be added studies that have been published in other countries, after Goffman and Freidson, by L. Albrecht, P. Abbot, M. Blaxter. If readers are not worried about getting lost in bibliography, they may consult the only one that exists with a historical perspective: G. Woodill, *Bibliographie signalétique, histoire des handicaps et inadaptations* (CTNERHI, 1988).

16. André Burguière, "L'Anthropologie historique," in *La Nouvelle Histoire*, ed. Jacques Le Goff (Éd. Complexes, 1988).

17. Claude Lévi-Strauss, *Anthropologie structurale deux* (Plon, 1973).

Chapter 2

1. For a collection of these texts, see Hans-Walter Wolff, ed., *Anthropologie de l'Ancien Testament* (Labor et Fides, 1974).

2. We should not neglect to associate with human defects the prohibitions concerning certain animals. The species that deviate from the definition of their kind are also distanced from sanctity. See, for example, D. Sperber, "Pourquoi les animaux parfaits, les hybrides et les monstres sont-il bons à penser symboliquement?" *L'Homme* 15 (1975).

3. Lev. 21.17–23, 22.21–22.

4. 2 Sam. 4.4.

5. For these various disabilities, see Deut. 15.21; Mal. 1.8; 2 Sam. 5.8; Num. 25.12.

6. *Encyclopedia Judaica*, (Macmillan and Keter, 1972) vol. 4, cols. 1081–84.

7. All these texts are found in the translation of the Qumran texts by A. Dupont-Sommer. See G. Marc Philonenko, "Une règle essénienne dans le Coran," *Semitica* 22 (1972).

8. Sura 24.60; and sura 48.

9. Luke 14.11–14.

10. Isa. 42.1–5, 49.1–6, 50.4–9, 52.13–53.12.

11. Girard, *La Violence et le sacré* and *Des choses cachées depuis la fondation du monde.* Only a very summary résumé is given here. See, for example, the journal *Esprit* 4 (April 1979).

12. The term *isotopy* is borrowed from the semiotics of A. J. Greimas. It designates a certain level that makes possible the coherence of a proposition. The isotopy guarantees the homogeneous character of a discourse, a message, a phrase. It is constituted by minimal characteristics that are

constant. For example, if I say, "He is an egghead," what ensures coherence, thanks to the features that are found in the context, is the isotopy of "intellectual activity," since we do not describe in this fashion a real physical head of such a shape. Or it may be a physiological isotopy that ensures homogeneity if the phrase were given a literal reading in another context; see, among others, Greimas, *Analyse sémiotique des textes,* Groupe d'Entrevernes (Presses Universitaires de Lyon, 1979).

13. See *Dictionnaire du Nouveau Testament,* ed. X. Leon-Dufour (Le Seuil, 1975), 453.

14. There are numerous passages in which Jesus is seen healing on the days of Sabbath: see, for example, Matt. 12.10–12; Mark 3.2–4; Luke 6.7–9.

15. It is quite evident that it is not my intention here to interpret Christianity and its New Testament foundations exclusively in a moral sense. My succinct phrasing is designed only to call attention to Jesus' humanity, if I may so speak, and the undeniable difficulty created by this perspective in relation to religions that had been established before him. It is true that the texts have a theological significance: Jesus is the healer, and the cures are above all signs—a sign that his disciples are capable of carrying on his work, a sign of the new world that has been heralded, a sign of spiritual healing, and also a sign of a world in which the poor have a position of honor. But beneath the theology the anthropologist discovers a conception of the sacral character of humanity itself and in particular of the weak (the Greek word most frequently used in the texts of the New Testament is *asthenia,* "infirmity, lack of strength").

Chapter 3

1. Marie Delcourt, *Stérilité mystérieuse et naissance maléfique dans l'Antiquité classique* (Liège, 1938). This is a very important book for our subject. I have chosen to base my comments on Delcourt, because among all the historians of classical Greek literature it is she who has best highlighted the problem of disability.

2. For this debate, see my discussion in connection with the myth of Oedipus and the interpretation of Girard.

3. In Rome, through the intermediary of augers, but this is the same thing in practice. Early Roman law required that the decision be taken, in the presence of five neighbors, by the "head of the family." Delcourt affirms that this is attested for all the Greek cities.

4. Delcourt cites all the texts that clearly indicate the religious character of the matter or that, under an overlay of other argumentation, still

let this first perspective show through: Sophocles, Plutarch, Plato, Aristotle, Denis of Halicarnassus, Seneca.

5. Similar remarks have been made for early Latin antiquity, among the Etruscans; R. Bloch, *Les Prodiges dans l'antiquité classique* (Presses Universitaires de France, 1963), 73. The transgression of biological laws is the expression of a serious divine menace, a reason for a dissolution of the pact between gods and humans, and must be expiated.

6. Contrary to the claims made in studies of the blind. For example, P. Villey, *L'Aveugle dans le monde des voyants*, Essai de Sociologie (Flammarion, 1927), writes that infants born blind were exposed. Pierre Henri, in his thesis *Les Aveugles et la société* (Paris: Presses Universitaires de France, 1958), relies on Villey. He admits, however, that the practice of exposure may perhaps not affect the blind (219). It would appear that we should not confuse the deformed (*amorphos* in Greek) with other disabilities such as blindness.

7. Cicero, *Tusculanes*, bk. 5, p. 38.

8. Aulus Gellius (120–175), *Attic Nights*, book 4, 2.

9. See, in this regard, Marcel Sendrail, *Histoire culturelle de la maladie* (Privat, 1980).

10. This is also true for Greece, but even more important is the threat of aberrancy.

11. Plato, *The Laws*, 11:10, 1079.

12. Dodds, *Les Grecs et l'irrationnel* (Flammarion, 1977); B. Simon, *Mind and Madness in Ancient Greece* (Cornell University Press, 1979); G. Rosen, *Madness and Society* (Harper and Row, 1969).

13. Plato, *Phaedrus*, 244A ff.

14. For madness addressed in therapeutic terms in antiquity, see the work of Jackie Peigeaud, *La Maladie de l'âme, étude sur la relation de l'âme et du corps dans la tradition médico-philosophique antique* (Les Belles Lettres, 1989); *Folie et cures de la folie chez les médecins de l'Antiquité gréco-romaine, La Manie* (Les Belles Lettres, 1987). See, too, Danièle Gourevitch, "Les Mots pour dire la folie en latin: À propos de Celse et Célius Aurélien," *L'Évolution Psychiatrique* 56 (1991).

15. Here, in addition to Dodds, the reader is referred to J.-P. Vernant and M. Detienne, for example, *Les Ruses de l'intelligence, la métis des Grecs* (Flammarion, 1974).

16. O. Jacob, "Les Cités grecques et les blessés de guerre," (Mélanges G. Glotz, 1932), 2:468.

17. Lysias, *Orationes*, ed. Th. Thalheim (Tübner, 1913), 24. At this period Lysias was a logographer, a kind of barrister and a master of rhetoric.

18. See, for example, Colette Astier, *Le Mythe d'Oedipe* (Armand Colin, 1974), a polysemic myth, since it deals with the question of power

and thus with politics, emotional questions, and thus family relations, the question of religion and thus the relationship with the divinity.

19. Delcourt, *Oedipe ou la Légende du Conquérant* (Liège, 1944). Her first chapter is entitled "The Exposed Infant." Her book was reiussed by Les Belles Lettres in 1981.

20. Ibid., 26f.

21. Lévi-Strauss, *Anthropologie structurale* (Plon, 1958; reprint, 1974), vol. 1, chap. 11.

22. The earlier book referred to here is *Stérilités mystérieuses et naissances maléfiques.* This citation from Delcourt, *Oedipe ou la légende,* 1.

23. Delcourt, *Stérilité mystérieuse.* Cypselus, tyrant of Corinth (697–625, B.C.E.), born of a lame (*labda*) mother but doubtless also lame himself; Paris, unlucky son of Priam, abandoned, rescued by shepherds, will ignite the Trojan War when he takes refuge in the city with Helen.

24. Delcourt, *Stérilité mystérieuse,* 21.

25. Nicole Belmont, "Les Rites de passage et la naissance: l'enfant exposé," *Dialogue* 127 (1995); reprinted from *Anthropologie et Société* 4, no. 2 (1980).

26. There are also other important figures of antiquity in the same situation as Oedipus. Romulus and Remus, the founders of Rome, are misfortune-bringing twins who are exposed but saved by the wolf that suckles them. At the very origins of Rome it is not prohibited to see deformity in full light!

27. No French word can be used in contrast to *différence. Identité* is ambiguous because it signifies not only the quality of a person but also the identical character of something. *Mêmeté* would be an unaesthetic neologism (although *sameness* is possible in English). Whence the necessity of using the Greek term *mimesis,* which is employed in philosophical discourse.

28. Girard, "Symétrie et dissymétrie dans le mythe d'Oedipe," *Critique* 249 (1968).

29. Again, it must be noted that such a statement privileges one version of the story, that of Sophocles. In some other versions Oedipus remains in Thebes and ends his days deep within the palace. But this version exists, and it is legitimate to seize on it.

30. The Gospel according to Mark 23. These served Girard in good stead in *Des Choses cachées depuis le commencement du monde* in support of his thesis of the Gospels as a revelation of the old victimizing mechanism.

31. I agree with Roland Barthes when he writes: "To interpret a text is not to give it sense (more or less based in it, more or less free); it is rather to appreciate the plurality of which it is composed," *S/Z* (Le Seuil, 1971),

11. All that I have done, even when structuring *one* reading, has been to add plurality to the myth of Oedipus. An individual reading is added to others, without renouncing them or destroying them.

32. Jean-Pierre Vernant, "Le Tyran boiteux, d'Oedipe à Périandre," in *Le Temps de la réflexion* (Éd. Gallimard, 1981; reprinted in J.-P. Vernant and P. Vidal-Naquet, *Oedipe et ses mythes,* Éd. Complexes, 1988).

33. Vernant, "Ambiguïté et renversement, Sur la structure énigmatique d'Oedipe-roi," in *Échanges et communications. Mélanges offerts à Claude Lévi-Strauss* 2 (1970): 1253–79; reprinted in J.-P. Vernant and P. Vidal-Naquet, *Oedipe et ses mythes,* Éd. Complexes, 1988).

34. Delcourt, *Héphaïstos ou la légende du magicien* (Les Belles Lettres, 1957), 131.

35. Delcourt, *Hermaphrodite, Mythes et rites de la bisexualité dans L'antiquité classique* (Presses Universitaires de France, 1958).

36. Ibid.

37. Ovid accounts for the origin of Hermaphrodite as precisely the result of the highly erotic union between a boy, born to Hermes and Aphrodite, and a nymph: at one moment their two bodies melt together.

38. Although this is not my topic, a word should be said about Hermaphrodite as figuring homosexuality. In no way do I wish to give the impression that homosexuality is being associated with the search for the same. Homosexual loves are differential, and it seems to me that Hermaphrodite quite exactly justifies this statement: he/she protects love affairs, all loves, for, at the very heart of the fusional quest that runs through all love, he/she shows its impossibility. This is no less true of homosexuality, which may take this course, than it is of heterosexuality, which is haunted by it as well.

Chapter 4

1. This is the view of Philippe Ariès, as expressed in a lecture given at the Semaine internationale de la réadaptation in March of 1981 at Strasbourg.

2. Claude Kappler, *Monstres, démons et merveilles à la fin du Moyen Âge* (Payot, 1980).

3. Without trying to be exhaustive in this regard, I would call attention to the most-read authors on this perspective: Michel Mollat, Jean-Louis Goglin, Jacques Heers, Guy Fourquier, Jean-Pierre Gutton.

4. J. Heers, *L'Occident aux XIVᵉ et XVIᵉ siècles aspects économiques et sociaux* (Presses Universitaires de France, 1973).

5. Jean Delumeau, *La Peur en Occident, XIVe–XVIIIe siècles* (Fayard, 1978), 131f.

6. Ibid., 410–14, conclusions. Thus, we can better understand that a François Charron, a Frenchman in Quebec, had the idea of requesting subsidies of Louis XIV in order to create workshops for the disabled in that distant province—and actually received them.

7. The Dominican Taddes Dini or the Franciscan Raymon Lulle. Cf. Michel Mollat, *Les Pauvres au Moyen Âge, étude sociale* (Hachette, 1978), 223–27.

8. Ibid., 40.

9. Ibid., 149.

10. J.-L. Goglin, *Les Misérables dans l'Occident médiéval* (Le Seuil, 1970).

11. Ibid., 68.

12. See specifically the selections from "The Battle between Carnival and Lent" that illustrate Goglin's book, But these motifs are to be found in many other paintings by Brueghel.

13. Goglin, *Les Misérables dans l'Occident Médiéval,* 159. It is in any case easy to understand that, when the intention to provide care did arise, the disabled—who were not ill in this era because the congenitally ill died—were excluded. On the contrary, in our era disabilities are attacked medically, and the disabled are once again cared for.

14. Ibid., 158.

15. There was a *ritual* of entrance into a leprosarium. François-Olivier Touati completed a very exhaustive study, "Lèpre, lépreux et léproseries dans la province ecclésiastique de Sens jusqu'au milieu du quatorzième siècle" (Ph.D. diss., 5 vols., Université-Panthéon-Sorbonne, Paris I, 1991). Part of this work, devoted exclusively to geography, was published under the title *Archives de la lèpre. Atlas des léproseries entre Loire et Marne au Moyen Âge* (CTHS, 1996).

16. Allard, Guy H., ed., *Aspects de la marginalité au Moyen Âge* L'Aurore, 1975), 42.

17. Ibid., 42.

18. Ibid., 75.

19. See, in this regard, the work by Jean Delumeau.

20. Allard, *Aspects,* 75. It must be admitted that the list of monstrosities is extremely varied. It goes from the giant or the pygmy to the cyclops, passing by way of the bearded lady and the hermaphrodite.

21. Maurice Lever, *Le Sceptre et la marotte. Histoire des fous de cour* (Fayard, 1983).

22. For this statement, see Kappler, "Le Monstre médiéval," *Revue d'Histoire et de Philosophie Religieuse de Strasbourg* 56 (1978). See, too,

Augustine's *The City of God*, 16:8; and David William, "Aspects du rôle médiateur des monstres," *Studies in Religion* 6 (1977), in which the author envisages the monster as "other" but also as representative of itself and as signifying God himself (there was an iconographical tradition of a monstrous Trinity). On monstrosity, see Claude Lecouteux, *Les Monstres dans la pensée médiévale européenne* (Presse de l'Université de Paris-Sorbonne, 1993).

23. Kappler, "Le Monstre médiéval."

24. Gilbert Dagron, *Naissance d'une capitale. Constantinople et ses institutions de 330 à 451* (Presses Universitaires de France, 1974).

25. See, for example, Homily 11 on the Acts of the Apostles, *Patrologie grecque*, vol. 60, cols. 96–98; cited in Dagron, *Naissance d'une capitale.*

26. Ibid., 509.

27. E. Patlagean, "Recherches sur les pauvres et la pauvreté dans l'empire romain d'Orient (IVe–VIIe siècles)" (Ph.D. diss., Lille, 1973).

28. The text is published in Michel Aubineau, "Biographie, vertu et martyre de notre Saint Père Zotikos, nourricier des pauvres," *Analecta Bollandiana* 93 (1975): 67–108. Dagron, from his perspective as historian, says that none of this is assured. But the unsure of the historian is not less sure for the historian of systems of thought and for the semiotician of cultures.

29. In this biography of Zotikos the vocabulary is very precise, specialized, and technical. Leprosy is designated by the word *lôbè* (maimed). We are then clearly in the register of deformity, disability.

30. The famous text of Saint Augustine is found in *The City of God*, 16:8.

31. Girard insists on this in his previously cited article on Oedipus.

32. J. Imbert, *Les Hôpitaux en droit canonique* (Vrin, 1947). The author notes that there is only a remote connection between the hospices and various actions undertaken in antiquity. The hospice is a creation of the Patristic period.

33. L. Lallemand, *Histoire de la charité*, vol. 3, *Le Moyen Âge* (A. Picard et fils, 1902), 126 ff.

34. I shall not deal with insanity in Middle Ages in this context. I refer readers to two books, the first is Muriel Laharie's *La Folie au Moyen Âge, XIe–XIIIe siècles*, preface by Jacques Le Goff (Le Léopard d'Or, 1991). This book perhaps overemphasizes insanity viewed as demonic possession. The Middle Ages were more tolerant than this book allows. This said, it is an extremely rich work, with an interesting bibliography. A second work is Jean-Marie Fritz, *Le Discours du fou au Moyen Âge, XIIe– XIIIe siècles, étude comparée des discours littéraire, juridique et théologique de la "folie"* (Presses Universitaires de France, 1992).

35. Imbert, *Les Hôpitaux en droit canonique,* 125.

36. Jacques le Goff, "Le Vocabulaire des catégories sociales chez saint François d'Assise et ses biographes du XIIIᵉ siècle" (1974), in *Ordres et Classes,* Colloque d'historie sociale (Mouton, 1957).

37. See, among others, Tudensz Manteuffel, *Naissance d'une hérésie, les adeptes de la pauvreté volontaire au Moyen Âge* (Mouton, 1963).

38. E. Longpré, *François d'Assise et son expérience spirituelle* (Beauchesne Éditeur, 1966).

39. Saint Francis of Assisi, *Documents: écrits et première biographie, rassemblés et présentés par Théophile Desbonnets et Damien Vorreux* (Éditions Franciscaines, 1968), 104. This work, now revised, contains the essential primary sources in a critical edition of great value.

40. One of his biographers shows that he replicated the ritual of entry into a leprosarium to typify his course of action (A. Fortini, *Francis of Assisi,* trans. Helen Moak [Crossroad, 1981]).

41. Paul Sabatier, *Études inédites sur saint François d'Assise* (Fischbacher, 1932), 158.

42. Omer Englebert, *Vie de Saint François d'Assise* (Albin Michel, 1952), 67. This author reiterates the statements of Thomas of Celano, the first biographer of Francis of Assisi.

43. See, for example, Michel Mollat, "Pauvres et pauvreté dans le monde médiéval," in *Povertà del Secolo XII* (E. Francesco d'Assisi, Società Internazionale di Studi Francesci, Assisi, 1975).

44. André Vauchez, "La Place de la pauvreté dans les documents hagiographiques à l'époque des Spirituels," in *Povertà del Secolo XII* (E. Francesco d'Assisi, Società Internazionale di Studi Francesci, Assisi, 1975).

45. Bronislaw Geremek, *Les Marginaux parisiens aux XIVᵉ et XVᵉ siècles* (Flammarion, 1976); *Truands et misérables dans l'Europe moderne (1350–1600)* (Gallimard/Juillard, 1980).

46. Ibid., 85.

47. Ibid., 98.

48. Ibid., 116.

49. Ibid., 164. Concerning the great division, which runs through the entire social question since the fourteenth century, between the beggars and the true poor, obliged to work, and the non-able-bodied poor, exempted from work and the object of assistance, see the masterful book of Robert Castel, *Les Métamorphoses de la question sociale, une chronique du salariat* (Fayard, 1995). One may profitably consult Philippe Sassier, *Du bon usage aux pauvres, histoire d'un thème politique, XVIᵉ–XXᵉ siècles* (Fayard, 1990). To fill out this view of the social issues, even if the topics discussed are different from those of Castel, it is rewarding to read

Bronislaw Geremek, *La Potence ou la pitié, l'Europe et les pauvres du Moyen Âge à nos jours* (Gallimard, 1987).

50. Geremek, *Truands et misérables,* 209.

51. Geremek, *Les Marginaux parisiens,* 223.

52. Ibid., 193–97.

53. Foucault, on the subject of lepers in the medieval period, writes of "a rigorous division which entails social exclusion but spiritual reintegration" (*Histoire de la folie, 10/18,* 18).

54. I cite as example Foucault, who in his lectures on the history of sexuality at the Collège de France in the winter of 1980–81 tries to show that the concepts of Christianity and paganism cannot be cited as grounds for the historical division. There is a system of aphrodisia, then one of the flesh . . . then of sexuality; this does not encompass the pagan/Christian distinction.

55. Without entirely espousing the point of view of Cornélius Castoriadis, it is still fairly clear that the ethical radicalism of the New Testament is such that "on this basis there is no society nor can there be one" (*La Montée de l'insignifiance, les carrefours du labyrinthe, IV* [Le Seuil, 1996], 217). It proved necessary for historical Christianity to make compromises.

Chapter 5

1. Ambroise Paré, *Des Monstres et prodiges,* ed. begun by Jean Céard (Droz, 1971).

2. Cf. the comments in Céard, *Des Monstres et prodiges.*

3. Sendrail, *Histoire culturelle de la maladie,* 317.

4. For an illuminating but brief discussion of Foucault's work, I refer to Michel de Certeau, "Le Noir soleil du langage," in *L'Absent de l'histoire* (Mame, 1973).

5. I owe a great deal to having read the vast work by Jacques Roger, *Les Sciences de la vie dans la pensée française du XVIIIe siècle, La génération des animaux de Descartes à l'Encyclopédie* (Armand Colin, 1963), re-edited with a preface by Claire Salmon-Bayet (Albin Michel, 1993).

6. Sylvain Régis, a Cartesian philosopher, 1632–1707.

7. Roger, *Les Sciences de la vie dans la pensée française,* 406.

8. Ibid., 418.

9. Jules Guérin, *Recherches sur les difformités congénitales chez les monstres, le foetus et l'enfant* (n.p., 1880). Guérin succeeds two great teratologists, the Geoffroy Saint Hilaires, father and son. The question of monstrosity from the seventeenth century onward has merited a separate study, which will be published shortly.

10. Saint Vincent de Paul was not the only one. Although the disciples of Saint Camille of Lellis were called the Ministers to the Disabled, the Camillians, such as the Frères de Saint-Jean de Dieu, like the Order of Saint Anthony of Viennois a bit before them, devoted themselves to the sick.

11. Certain historians, such as Ariès, believe that many disabled children disappeared "accidentally," by smothering or by "falling" into a well or in other ways. These historians base their claims on the edicts of bishops prohibiting that children sleep in the parental bed. These edicts do not seem to have been prompted by (psychologically alert!) principles of child rearing but by the desire to eliminate camouflaged infanticide.

12. B. Dompnier, *Le XVIIᵉ siècle français: Quand tout pouvoir se nommait charité,* Lumière et Vie 28, no. 142 (1979).

13. Arthur Loth, *Saint Vincent de Paul et sa mission sociale* (D. Dumoulin, 1880), 177 ff.

14. Pierre Coste, *Le Grand saint du grand siècle. Monsieur Vincent* (Desclée de Brouwer, 1934), 726.

15. The affiliation between the Maison du Nom de Jésus and the Hôpital Général has been identified and posited by L. Lallemand, *Histoire de la charité* (A. Picard et fils, 1902), 4:400 ff.

16. Quoted in Dompnier, *Le XVIIᵉ siècle franĉais,* 10.

17. L. Lallemand does not hesitate to make this claim at the beginning of volume 5. More certain, however, is the fact that the movement toward a laicization of charity was furthered by the Reformation.

18. For the differences in approach of these two schools, Vives on the one hand and Soto on the other, see Lallemand, *Histoire de la charité,* vol. 4.

19. Founded by Cardinal de la Rochefoucauld.

20. *Oeuvres complètes de Vincent de Paul* (Ed. Coste, n.d.), 10:339.

21. For this whole question, see Robert Chaboche, "Le Sort des militaires invalides avant 1674," in *Les Invalides, trois siècles d'histoire* (n.p., 1974).

22. Again from the work quoted earlier, *Les Invalides,* see the essay by Colonel Henri de Buttot, "Les Compagnies détachées des Invalides."

23. This is emphasized by A. Soubiran, "Le Service de santé des Invalides," in *Les Invalides.*

24. Col. H. de Buttot, "La Vie aux Invalides sous le règne de Louis XIV," in *Les Invalides.*

25. We should note just how successful Turgot and the philanthropic movement, of which he was the standard bearer, were in creating a grand doctrine of social assistance. The French Revolution and its Committee on Begging, of which Larochefoucauld-Liancourt was the president, were

their heirs. The question of the disabled among the larger social issues of the eighteenth century deserves much more than the few pages devoted to it here. Readers are referred, while awaiting the appearance of a study in progress, to Castel, "Les Métamorphoses"; see, too, Alan Forrest, *La Révolution française et les pauvres* (Perrin, 1986).

26. I have this information from Robert Heller, "Educating the Blind in the Age of Enlightenment: Growing Pains of a Social Service," *Medical History* 23 (1979).

27. Jean-Jacques Rousseau, for example, worked toward the creation of an establishment for the disabled in Switzerland.

28. Roger, *Les Sciences*, 598.

29. Jean-Pierre Peter, *Le Grand rêve de l'ordre médical, en 1770 et aujourd'hui*, Autrement Éditions, No. 4. 75–76, *Guérir pour normaliser.*

30. Ibid., 188.

31. Robert Castel, *L'Ordre psychiatrique, l'âge d'or de l'aliénisme* (Editions de Minuit, 1976).

32. Since 1962 studies on the period and the personalities of Valentin Haüy and the abbé de l'Épée have expanded. See in the appended bibliography the works by Bézagu-Deluy, the writings of the abbé, Harlan Lane, Zina Weygand. The reader may also refer to *Les acquis de la révolution française pour les personnes handicapées de 1789 à nos jours* (proceedings of a colloquium held at the Université de Paris X-Nanterre on the bicentenary of the French Revolution, March 22, 1989; coordinated by Pierre Turpin).

33. Louis Braille (1809–52) did not realize his invention alone and in a single stroke. Haüy had explored the use of conventional writing in relief ("waffled," as it was called in French); Barbier de la Serre (after Father Lana in 1670) had the idea of raised dots. The genius of Louis Braille lay in simplicity and systematization, which made his writing and reading system truly popular.

34. Pierre Villey, *Le Monde des aveugles*, rev. ed. (Corti J., 1984).

35. Pierre Villey, *L'Aveugle dans le monde des voyants, Essai de sociologie* (Flammarion, 1927), 315.

36. I would recall here that I exclude insanity during the previous century from my study, given the numerous works that have been written on the subject. I am speaking of (re)education institutions for the purpose of schooling and vocational training and not of orthopedic institutions or those for medical care (see later discussion for such establishments).

37. First article of a bill: "The National Assembly declares that it ranks among the most sacred duties of the nation assistance to the poor of all ages and in all circumstances of life and that provision shall be made. . . ."

38. The legislation and the general spirit of the Revolution and of the

nineteenth century are gathered in an unjustly neglected work: Fernand Charoy 1906, "L'Assistance aux vieillards, infirmes et incurables en France de 1789 à 1905" (Ph.D. diss., Faculty of Law, University of Paris, 1906).

39. Expenses were to be borne by the family at first and, in the event of lack of resources, by a *national* assistance program, not a municipal or local one. "Aid to the class of unfortunates is the responsibility of the State, like the payment of public servants, like the costs of the Church" (Third Report of the Committee).

40. Castel, *L'Ordre psychiatrique,* 44 ff.

41. Ibid., 49.

42. Laws of 16 Vendémiaire and 7 Frimaire, 1795.

43. Beggar cells existed during the ancien régime (before the Revolution) and would be recreated during the empire. With the pretext and intention of helping, they amounted to incarceration. F. Charoy writes: "The result was that the aged and the disabled, unable to live without asking for alms, were destined to be arrested, condemned, and finally find asylum in the prisons" (*L'Assistance aux vieillards,* 61).

44. As readers will note, in 1962 I relied principally on the works of Foucault and Castel. Today, after the impressive work of Marcel Gauchet and Gladys Swain, I would compare the institutions created by the older Pinel with that of Haüy and the abbé de l'Épée and would challenge the thesis of the latter part of Foucault's *Histoire de la folie à l'âge classique,* for Gauchet and Swain have clearly seen that a democratic anthropology, with a requirement for all-out inclusion, had been at work for at least two centuries.

45. Castel, *L'Ordre psychiatrique,* 162.

46. The law of 1838 was not repealed until the passage of a new law on internment on June 27, 1990. But the new law is still very similar to that of 1838, save in the detail of the departmental commission for the control of hospitalization. See Jacques Postel, "La Nouvelle loi française sur l'internement," *Nouvelle histoire de la psychiatrie,* 446 ff.

47. See the brochure (perhaps by Vincent Duval) entitled *Institut orthopédique,* dated 1850. In the same vein are the *Établissement orthopédique* of Dr. Sauveur Henri-Victor (Bouvier, 1853); and *Notice sur l'Institut orthopédique et gymnastique* of Jean-Charles Pravaz (n.p., 1863).

48. The same V. Duval wrote an *Aperçu sur les principales difformités du corps humain* (published privately, 1833), which he addressed to the General Council of Hospitals of Paris. There he furnished abundant proof that the cripples of the hospitals originated in the working (and subproletariat) class.

49. In 1861 the first establishment was put up at Berck-sur-Mer, built of wood but as a permanent structure, completed in 1869, with 500 beds, more than 80 infirmary beds, plus another small hospital of 100 beds. In 1860 Forges-les-Bains had 112 beds.

50. A discussion of the different extension beds that were in use can be found in Charles-André Maisonable's defence of his own in the *Journal Clinique,* where he offers a "collection of observations on the deformities to which the human body is susceptible at various stages of life, and in particular what relates in general to mechanics and the instruments employed in surgery" (Paris, 1825).

51. Henri-Victor Bouvier, *Électricité médicale* (n.p., 1856).

52. H.-V. Bouvier, *Étude historique et médicale sur l'usage des corsets* (1853).

53. For these problems related to the evolution of ideas about the body and techniques for it, see G. Vigarello, *Le Corps redressé* (J.-P. Delarge, 1978). For the present discussion, see "L'inversion des machines," 142 ff. The analysis of musculature, both dynamic and mechanically deconstructed, appears in the nineteenth century and led to the biomechanics of today.

54. Albert Montheuil, *La Charité privée à l'étranger* (n.p., 1898).

55. The society assumed responsibility for the sales of the goods produced. It bore the costs of products that it paid for but could not place with the public.

56. Montheuil, *La Charité privée,* 185–91.

57. The National Industrial Home for Crippled Boys; and the Cripples' Home and Industrial School for Girls.

58. Readers will have noted that I have scarcely said anything about the education and training of the retarded, and yet this is the sphere that has been most and best studied. It is then essential to name the primary reference works: Capul, Gateaux-Mennecier, Raynaud, Boivin, Diederich.

Chapter 6

1. The French term *mutilé* figured in the first juridical text passed even before the end of the war, on January 2, 1918: "Vocational rerehabilitation and national office of the war maimed and medically discharged." The phrase *invalide (de guerre)* was also current and carried its own semantic charge.

2. Since 1962 a great deal of scholarly work has been undertaken on the history of the war wounded and its impact on the whole of French society; the principal architect is Jean-François Montès, in particular with

his dissertation in the social sciences, "Infirmités et invention de l'action sociale, sens et convergence de leurs histoires" (Institut Catholique de Paris [IES], 1991).

3. The reference work for the war wounded and veterans is Antoine Prost, *Les Anciens combattants et la société française, 1914–1939,* 3 vols. (Presses de la Fondation Nationale des Sciences Politiques, n.d.). I regret that the aspect that I am emphasizing should not have received more concentrated attention there. On the other hand, this book shows that the origin of all work of rehabilitation is to be found in the problems raised by the redeployment and compensation of impaired veterans.

4. This word (*réintegrer*) became official and current, in parallel with the word *réinsertion* (reinsertion), which is not found in French dictionaries. In France the latter unfortunately caught on better than the former.

5. I have emphasized this point on several occasions, for example in "Handicap et exclusion, la construction sociale du handicap," in *L'Exclusion, l'état des savoirs,* ed. Serge Paugam (Éd. la Découverte, 1996).

6. A law was passed in July 1893 to create cost-free medical assistance. The same vocabulary recurs in the law of June 27, 1904, concerning child assistance and that of July 14, 1905, on the disabled and incurable elderly. For further legislation (with the exception of sociojudicial legislation concerning childhood, such as the law of July 22, 1912), we must look to the period after the war to find the continuation of juridical work in this vein.

7. J. Verdes-Leroux, *Le Travail social* (Éd. de Minuit, 1978).

> Social assistance, in thus constituting itself, designates and isolates its target, *the urban working class,* which is then distinguished from the mass of "those who can be helped." That is to say, social assistance abandons to public welfare and to charity the poor and other 'unredeemables' who make up an unproductive and, for the aid program, a politically innocuous group. The opposition is no longer between the poor and the rich, but between the proletariat and the capitalists. (16)

8. My stance is above all inspired by the book by François Ewald, *L'État providence* (Grasset et Fasquelle, 1986). To complete this view of the history of the evolution that runs from the infirm of an earlier age to the disabled worker, see Pascal Doriguzzi, *L'Histoire politique du handicap, de l'infirme au travailleur handicapé* (L'Harmattan, 1994).

9. Verdes-Leroux, *Le Travail social,* 41, for example. This author makes a very sharp distinction at this point.

10. See the appendix.

11. See chapter 2 and note 12.

12. Law of June 30, 1975: Law on the counseling of disabled persons (see the app.).

13. In my mind these other discourses are typified by the law concerning adult incompetents of January 1968. This text, dealing with mental illness, dismantles the notorious law of 1838 on the insane. Internment is rescinded, since the mentally ill can now be put in the care of a guardian.

14. See this idea in Roger Gentis, "Demain les autres," *En Marge, l'Occident et ses autres* (Aubier, 1978).

15. Michel Foucault, *Histoire de la folie à l'âge classique* (Plon, 1961; reprint, Éd. Gallimard, 1972); and 10/18

16. See the work of T. Szasz, one of whose books is entitled *L'Âge de la folie* (PUF, 1978).

17. For this shift, effected in the nineteenth century, see Castel, *L'Ordre psychiatrique.*

18. These financial reasons (and I shall return to them later) should be taken for what they are: pretexts. The criticism of heightened costs is a screen and a trap, because money is not as lacking as authorities would have it (a slightly different budgetary option would be enough or even, at times, a change in allocations). It is clear that social policy is not driven by financial considerations. There is no money because they want social policy of a certain kind, not the other way around.

19. Here, too, I would agree with the analysis of Verdes-Leroux at the end of her work concerning the book by R. Lenoir, *Les Exclus* (Le Seuil, 1974), but I would also disagree. She has clearly seen the book's effort at *intimidation* in order to further the initiative of social defense. I am less convinced of its function to concentrate the dominant and disperse the dominated.

20. This is how I understand the contradiction between the principles established by the law of 1975 and the very numerous decrees for its implementation. The retrograde effects of these decrees almost all have to do with specialized action: penalties imposed on the most productive earners in the sheltered workplaces, reduction in training time in the specialized centers, delays in setting up counseling programs, etc.

21. Laws of 1924 and 1957 on the quota of disabled. Cf. the appendix. To this should be added the law of July 10, 1987.

22. A full analysis of the passage from the Great Confinement to alienation, starting in the revolutionary period and leading to the law of 1838, which will dominate the regulation of mental illness for a century, has been very pertinently made by Castel, *L'Ordre psychiatrique.* His book shows three waves since the Revolution (despite multiple movements of ebb and flow): the era of Pinel, when the dominant idea was more a social

than a medical operation; the era of the law, which synthesized the social and the medical; and the present critical era, which questions the need for internment.

23. This is clearly the case for persons with cerebral palsy (CP), who, frequently without control over either their gestures or speech, are considered feeble-minded . . . and risk becoming so (at least "falsely") in the sense that, put in the company of senile persons or those with mental disorders, nothing is done to develop their ability. The symptomatology that was earlier prevalent (e.g., Pinel in the nineteenth century) continues to find expression in widespread images: severe physical affliction is assimilated to mental derangement.

24. This claim will emerge on its own in what follows, but it should be clear by this time to the reader that the forms of social treatment of mental cases resemble those of the physical cases.

25. La Société des Croix-Marines in 1935.

26. Castel, *L'Ordre psychiatrique*, 266 ff.

27. The following, in fact, appear to have been more decisive: the psychoanalytic movement, on the one hand, and the ill-named "antipsychiatry," on the other (in the United States; in England, with Laing and Cooper; in France, with M. Mannoni, etc.).

28. The French establishments for maladjusted youth (juvenile delinquents, troubled youth; both mental and social factors are envisaged) are: the IMPP (medico-psychological educational institutions), frameworks for counseling; the IMP (medico-educational institutions), frameworks to receive patients during the schooling period; the IMPRO (medico-vocational institutions), structures that aim at vocational redeployment for adolescents. For adults there are either temporary structures, often called retraining centers, or more long-lasting arrangements, such as centers for assistance through employment, which have both residential and day clients.

29. As, for example, persons with low or very low IQs, with Down's syndrome, in contrast to schizophrenic, depressive, or paranoid persons.

30. It would be tiresome to list the hundreds of associations that sprang up after 1945. The first, which were trendsetting, were begun in the 1930s. This is true of both France and the rest of western Europe.

31. Besides the associations for those with sensory impairment that dated from the nineteenth century, the first rehabilitation schools were created by the National Office for the War Maimed (Office National des Mutilés). In the civil world Berck was the cradle. Here it seems that the very first persons to have had the will to recreate an integral place for the disabled in society, in particular through the medium of work, were Madeleine Rivard and Maurice Henry.

32. The League for the Adaptation of the Physically Impaired to Work (La ligue pour l'adaptation du diminué physique au travail [Ladapt]); the autobiography of S. Fouché, *J'espérais un grand espoir* (Du Cerf, 1981).

33. We may name Suzanne Fouché, founder of Ladapt; André Trannoy, founder of APF; and Madeleine Rivard, founder of Auxilia. In January 1995 the society Alter, for the history of deficiencies, maladjustments, disabilities . . . organized an important conference on the relationships between the associations and the state in the construction of disability as a recognized field. The proceedings are being edited and will be published by Presses Universitaires de Rennes.

34. Unapei now includes in its programs not only very accessible centers for Aid through Work but also has the objective of vocational training and employment in the ordinary sector for those who were classed as developmentally retarded (mildly and severely). There is a great ambiguity in this kind of association, between the discourse of integration and the administrative, and parental, discourse that protects these institutions, already protected in other ways!

35. See Christian Delacampagne, *Les Figures de l'oppression* (Presses Universitaires de France, 1977).

36. I remember a discussion concerning the logo for an association, an interregional grouping for the reintroduction of the disabled into the workforce that stemmed from the initiative of a number of companies employing disabled labor. The logo that was finally chosen was an abstraction with different shapes and surfaces combining into a hexagon, in order to indicate unity in difference. The graphic was interesting but nonetheless concealing: there was no longer any allusion to *mal*-formation.

37. I would insist on two of my studies, which might usefully have been substituted for the 1962 text: *De la métaphore au modèle: l'anthropologie du handicap Cahiers Ethnologiques* (Bordeaux) 13; and "Handicap, handicapé," *Handicap et Inadaptation. Fragments pour une histoire. Notions et acteurs* (Alter, 1996).

38. My perspective has been the object of widespread discussion and elaboration. See, for example, the number of *Sciences Sociales et Santé* listed in the bibliography, in which the authors cite my work on almost every page.

39. The year 1981 was declared the International Year of the Handicapped.

40. A technical commission for counseling and vocational redeployment (Cotorep) for adults, particularly as concerns the right to work and to training; departmental (regional) commission for special education (CDES) for the younger disabled.

41. Lévi-Strauss, *Le Totémisme aujourd'hui* (Presses Universitaires de France, 1969).

42. Jacques Léonard, *La Médicine entre les pouvoirs et les savoirs, histoire intellectuelle et politique de la médicine française au XIXᵉ siècle* (Aubier-Montaigne, 1981).

43. Ph. Saint-Martin, in *Handicaps, "Handicaper,"* proceedings of the colloquium organized by the French Communist Party, June 17–19, 1977 (Éd. Sociales, 1978).

44. This statement must be qualified to take into account the most recent initiatives. For example, without being in the least exhaustive: the SSESD, now the SESSAD (special education and home care services), which permit the child to stay in a school environment; or, for adults, the OPI, boards for reentry, placement, and support on the ordinary labor market. But what I am looking at here is the importance of work "on and with" civil society, which is still unfunded. See my article "Un Acteur trop absent, la société civile," *Communications et handicaps* (Conservatoire National des Arts et Métiers, 1988).

45. See the demonstration of this thesis by B. Lory in the study, *La Politique d'action sociale* (Éd. Privat, 1975).

46. Readers may be surprised that I have retained these lines that seem more applicable to 1962. For the moment it is not really a question of cutting off this positive discrimination in the area of social coverage. Even if it is not certain that everything will remain in place, the 150 billion odd francs that disability annually costs the French nation is not disputed by anyone. Paying remains a way of getting ourselves off the hook in the face of a problem as intolerable as it is incriminating. We have an indication, although the sums here in question do not go to social action, in the fact that about 50 percent of employers who are under the obligation of a quota of 6 percent of disabled workers in their workforce, according to the legislation of 1987, contribute to a fund (AGEFIPH). One can always retort that there are 50 percent who do not contribute and that those who do contribute do not always do so to the full limit of their obligation, either because they already have a certain percentage or because they get off, in part, by providing employment in the form of sheltered workshops. This is not really relevant to these concerns, since the half-full or half-empty bottle is a false problem.

47. Patrick Fugeyrollas, "Normalité et corps différents, regard sur l'intégration sociale des handicapés physiques," *Anthropologie et Société* (Montréal, Université de Laval) 2, no. 2. Christian Delacampagne writes: "What I want to show is that exclusion hides a recuperation ploy. That internment is much more warehousing than rejection, more a new divi-

sion (within the social space) than an expulsion. In short, at the moment when they thought themselves excluded, when they in fact were, the insane were also at the same time *included,* but in a new place, in new networks and in such a fashion as to satisfy the essential functions of the social body in its entirety" (*Les Figures de l'oppression* [Presses Universitaires de France, 1977], 79).

48. Here, too, it may be thought that my analysis is dated. It is certain that the attention of social critics has been considerably displaced and that the question of power has recently been a bit neglected. Moreover, physicians have continuously seen their reputation diminished. Yet within the commissions (CDES, Cotorep) at the heart of the relevant research bodies, in the official identification of disability, etc., doctors remain dominant. It is too soon to say that an analysis of the importance of their power is a dead subject.

49. Within the counseling commissions (official instances). Within all the institutions, even those with vocational or educational goals. Within the preparatory and follow-up teams (also official instances, created in France by the law of 1975).

50. Here I am thinking of the Henri-Poincaré Hospital in Garches, for example, and of Professor A. Grossiord, whose inspiration it was. See the book by J.-P. Held, *A Grossiord. La Médecine de rééducation* (Flammarion, 1981), introduction.

51. My chief reference here is to Foucault, *La Naissance de la clinique,* 2d ed. (Presses Universitaires de France, 1980).

52. The Raymond Poincaré Hospital in Garches, the Center for Therapy and Rehabilitation in Kerpape (Lorient), the establishments at Berck-Plage, etc. Each counts hundreds of clients.

53. François Fourquet and Léon Murard, *Histoire de la psychiatrie du secteur* (Éd. Recherches, 1980). This book, composed of interviews with the major figures who established sectorization, does not treat the present subject, since it is entirely centered on insanity. But we see a bit of Sivadon, Aujaleu, Oury, in physical medicine, if only through the link—which was particularly the work of Aujaleu—with tuberculosis. By the very force of things tuberculosis, the discovery of its causes and its prevention, dictated the first guidelines for sectorization.

54. Physiotherapy, balneotherapy, ergotherapy, etc.

55. I regret not having developed this point with regard to the relationship between the school and disability, the more so because the Italian example is very stimulating. I am obliged to refer to the most significant studies: Lucia De Anna 1996, "L'intégration scolaire des enfants handicapés en Italie," *Cahiers du CTNERHI* 72. See, too, Pierre Bonjour and

Michèle Lapeyre, *Handicaps et vie scolaire, l'intégration différenciée* (Chronique Sociale, 1994).

56. Admittedly, tendencies differ. In the Netherlands specific protected employment has been developed; in Denmark there has been a push toward nonemployment; in Quebec authorities balked at the idea of a specialized training system for the disabled. For comparisons within Europe, see "Handicaps et inadaptations. Le travail des personnes handicapées à l'heure européene," *Cahiers du CTNERHI* 65–66 (January–June 1995). This study is very full and features the most authoritative authors and an ample bibliography.

57. Training in the trades and crafts has practically disappeared; training for careers in the leisure industry or the arts does not exist, with the exception of some openings for blind musicians.

58. Although there are equivalents in other countries, a very large sector of industrial education in France is administered by an agency accountable to the Ministry of Labor: the Association pour la formation professionnelle des adultes (AFPA), an association for the vocational training of adults. Even in the case when technical training is under the Ministry of Education (or its equivalent), it is the employers who are in control. This is even more true of the private technical schools, whether or not they are directly linked to specific companies.

59. The word *détour* is borrowed from Raynaud, *L'éducation spécialisée.* The author attempts to resurrect both the program of Binet and Simon and special education in a democratic sense. It is not my purpose to make a judgment, although it seems to me that the author's demonstration is forced, and he forgets that these detours are often without a way back, even if the true sense of the word is a route to return to the normal itinerary. These detours, often long and sometimes without exit, seem to me typical of what Robert Murphy, in *The Body Silent* (Holt, 1987), analyzes as the modern status of the disabled: a threshold situation, perpetually liminal.

60. Henri-Jacques Stiker, *Culture brisée, culture à naître* 76 ff.

61. The drafting of the law of 1976 in France was exemplary: each institution was consulted after a fashion, but there was no collective effort to establish a common front. A congress was held (under the auspices of a federation named FAGERH) . . . but after the law had been passed!

62. Bearing witness to this is Robert Buron, a rehabilitation pioneer who early saw the political dimension. A former patient at Berck-Plage, he went on to a career in politics. See the opening pages of his book *Par goût de la vie* (Éd. du Cerf, 1973).

63. We know that the concept of production remains fundamental to

critical social thought since Marx but also that this concept is itself very ideological. See Jean Baudrillard, *Le Mirroir de la production* (Castermann, 1973).

64. See Claude Alzon, *Femme boniche, femme potiche* (Cahiers Libres, Maspéro, 1973), in which the author exposes this aspect very well, as seen through the eyes of Marxist theory.

65. I return here to this concept from semiotics, deriving from A.-J. Greimas, which I have already defined more explicitly in my second chapter (n. 12).

66. Reference must be made here to Georges Canguilhem, *Le Normal et le pathologique* (Presses Universitaires de France, 1966). The author exposes the arbitrariness of thinking of the pathological from the perspective of the normal, while in fact the pathological is a version of the normal, is "another normality" (135). "Objectively, we can define only varieties or differences, without positive or negative value" (153). But my analysis is located in another register.

67. *Seme:* the minimum unit of sense. Each word, each package of meanings is made up of smaller units. For example, the word *head* comprises various semes: superiority, extremity, representativity, etc.

68. I have purposely not written *Christian system,* since, if one system or another may have prevailed during what we call Judaism or paganism or Christianity, it is not a given that the system is Jewish, pagan, or Christian. The history of systems of redistribution is different from those of religion!

69. We have seen this among the Jews of the Old Testament: the priest identifies and decides on the disability and its clean or unclean character.

70. See, for example, among other works, *Le Sale espoir* by Annie Lauran (L'Harmattan, 1981).

71. See, for example, the Movement for the Defense of the Disabled in France, Carrefour Handicapé à Québec, etc.

Epilogue

1. We must hear and listen attentively to the lives of those who have suffered so much from such uprooting and specialized environments. See Aisha, *Décharge publique, les emmurés de l'assistance* (Maspéro, 1979).

2. The lines of my thought connect, to a great extent, with the book, *Vivre dans la différence, handicap et réadaptation dans la société d'aujourd'hui,* ed. Claude Veil (Privat, 1982).

3. The directions for thought and action that are proposed here can be

deflected from their true course. If they were taken as a pretext to reduce support for existing institutions in order to return to a less expensive form of aid, their objective would have been betrayed.

4.   I allude here to the debate promoted by the journal *Esprit* concerning thinkers like Louis Dumont (*Homo aequalis,* [Gallimard, 1977]), Pierre Rosanvallon, ("État providence et société solidaire," *Esprit,* nos. 7–8 [1978]), and all that followed, both from the Frankfurt school and from Castoriadis or C. Lefort.

Selected Bibliography

Abbot, P. *Towards a Social Theory of Handicap.* Ph.D., diss., CNAA / Thames Polytechnic, London, 1982.

Albrecht, Gary L. *The Sociology of Physical Disability and Rehabilitation.* University of Pittsburgh, 1976.

———. *The Disability Business: Rehabilitation in America.* Sage Publications, 1992.

Allard, Guy H., ed. *Aspects de la marginalité au Moyen Âge.* L'Aurore, 1975.

Althabe, Gérard. "Ethnologie du contemporain, anthropologie de l'ailleurs." In *L'état des sciences sociales en France.* Éditions la Découverte, 1986.

Assouly-Piquet, Collette, and Francette Berthier-Vittoz. *Regards sur le handicap.* Preface by Monique Schneider. Épi, 1994.

Avan Louis, Michel Fardeau, and Henri-Jacques Stiker. *L'homme réparé, artifices, victoires, défis.* Éd. Gallimard, 1988.

Baudrillard, Jean. *La transparence du mal, essai sur les phénomènes extrêmes.* Galilée, 1990.

Belmont, Nicole. "Les rites de passage et la naissance, l'enfant exposé." *Dialogue,* no. 127 (1995). Reprinted from *Anthropologie et Sociétés* 4, no. 2 (1980).

Bézagu-Deluy, Maryse. *L'abbé de L'Épée, instituteur gratuit des sourds et muets, 1712–1789.* Seghers, 1990.

Biraben, Jean-Noël. *Les hommes et la peste en France et dans les pays européens et méditerranéens.* Vol. 1: *La peste dans l'histoire.* Paris-La Haye, 1975. Vol. 2: *Les hommes face à la peste.* Paris-La Haye, 1976.

Blanc, Alain. *Les handicapés au travail, analyse sociologique d'un dispositif d'insertion professionnelle.* Dunod, 1995.

Blaxter, M. *The meaning of disability: a sociological study of disability.* Heinemann, 1976.

Bloch, R. *Les prodiges dans l'Antiquité classique.* PUF, 1963.

Boiral, Pierre, and Jean-Pierre Brouat. *Les représentations sociales de la folie.* Coop. Recherche, 1984.
Boivin, Jean-Pierre. "De la genèse de l'éducaiton spéciale à l'invention des enfants handicapés mentaux." Ph.D. diss., Department of Sociology (advisor, Robert Castel), Université Paris VIII, 1988.
Bonjour, Pierre, and Michele Lapeyre. *Handicaps et vie scolaire, l'intégration différenciée.* Chronique Sociale, 1994.
Bourdieu, Pierre. *Questions de sociologie.* Éd. de Minuit, 1984.
Burguière, André. "L'Anthropologie historique." In *La Nouvelle histoire,* ed. Jacques Le Goff. Éd. Complexes, 1988.
Canguilhem, Georges. "La Monstruosité et le monstrueux." *Diogène,* no. 40 (1962).
———. *Le Normal et le pathologique.* PUF, 1966.
Capul, Maurice. *Abandon et marginalité, les enfants placés sous l'Ancien Régime.* Preface by Michel Serres. Éd. Privat, 1989.
———. *Infirmité et hérésie, les enfants placés sous l'Ancien Régime.* Éd. Privat, 1990.
Caspar, Philippe. *Le Peuple des silencieux, une histoire de la déficience mentale.* Éd. Fleurus, 1994.
Castel, Robert. *Les Métamorphoses de la question sociale, une chronique du salariat.* Fayard, 1995.
———. "De l'indigence à l'exclusion, la désaffiliation. Précarité du travail et vulnérabilité relationnelle." In *Face à l'exclusion. Le modèle français,* ed. J. Donzelot. *Esprit* (1991).
———. *La Gestion des risques, de l'anti-psychiatrie à l'après-psychanalyse.* Éd. de Minuit, 1981.
———. *L'Ordre psychiatrique, l'âge d'or de l'aliénisme.* Éd. de Minuit, 1976.
Certeau, Michel de. *L'Absent de l'histoire.* Éd. Mame, 1973.
———. "L'Opération historique." In *Faire de l'histoire,* vol. 1; Nouveaux problèmes, ed. J. Le Goff and Pierre Nora. Éd. Gallimard, 1974.
Charoy, Fernand. *L'Assistance aux vieillards, infirmes et incurables en France de 1789 à 1905.* Ph.D. diss., Faculté de Droit, Paris, 1906.
Chauvière, Michel. *Enfance inadaptée: l'héritage de Vichy.* Éd. de l'Atelier / Éd. Ouvrières, 1980.
Chesler, M. A. "Ethnocentrism and Attitudes toward Disabled Persons. In *Rehabilitation Research and Practice Review* (1965). Reprinted from J. Hanks, "The Physically Disabled in Certain Non-Occidental Societies." *Journal of Social Issues* 4 (1948).
———. "Classer les assistés (1980–1914)." *Cahiers de la Recherche sur le travail social,* no. 19 (1990).
Classification internationale des handicaps: déficiences, incapacités, dés-

avantages, un manuel de classification des conséquences des maladies, published in English as *International Classification of Impairments, Disabilities, and Handicaps: A Manual of Classification Relating to the Consequences of Disease.* World Health Organization, 1980. Reprint, CTNERHI-INSERM, 1988.

Collée, Michel, and Claude Quétel. *Histoire des maladies mentales.* PUF and QSJ, 1987.

Dagron, Gilbert. *Naissance d'une capitale, Constantinople et ses institutions de 330 à 451.* PUF, 1974.

De Anna, Lucia. "L'intégration scolaire des enfants handicapées en Italie." *Les Cahiers du CTNERHI,* no. 72 (October–December 1996).

———. "De l'infirmité au handicap, jalons historiques." *Cahiers du CTNERHI,* no. 50 (April–June 1990).

Delacampagne, Christian. *Les Figures de l'oppression.* PUF, 1977.

Delcourt, Marie. *Stérilité mystérieuse et naissance maléfique dans l'antiquité classique.* Liège, 1938. Reprint, Les Belles Lettres, 1986.

———. *Œdipe ou la légende du conquérant.* Liège, 1944. Reprint, Les Belles Lettres, 1981.

Deleuze, Gilles. *Foucault.* Éd. de Minuit, 1986.

Delumeau, Jean. *La peur en Occident, XIVᵉ–XVIIIᵉ siècles.* Fayard, 1978.

Diederich, Nicole. *Les Naufragés de l'intelligence.* Syros, 1990.

Diogène. September 1996. Ed. Aude de Saint Loup.

Dodds, E. R. *The Greeks and the Irrational.* Trans., Flammarion, 1977.

Donzelot, J., ed. *Face à l'exclusion. Le modèle franĉais.* Éd. Esprit, 1991.

Doriguzzi, Pascal. *L'histoire politique du handicap, de l'infirme au travailleur handicapé.* L'Harmattan Éd., 1994.

Droz, J., ed. *Histoire générale du socialisme.* 2 vols. PUF, 1972–74.

Duby, Georges, and Michelle Perrot. *Histoire des femmes en Occident.* Plon. 5 vols. n.d.

Dupaquier, Jean, ed. *Histoire de la population française.* PUF, 1990.

Ellenstein, Jean, ed. *Histoire mondiale des socialismes.* Armand Colin, 1984.

de l'Épée, abbé Charles-Michel. *La véritable manière d'instruire les sourds et muets, confirmée par une longue expérience.* Corpus des œuvres de philosophie en langue française. Fayard, 1984.

Ewald, François. *L'État Providence.* Grasset, 1986.

Farrell, G. *The History of Blindness.* Harvard University Press, 1956.

Forest, Alan. *La Révolution française et les pauvres,* Oxford, 1981. Reprint, Perrin, 1986.

Foucault, Michel. *Histoire de la folie à l'âge classique.* Plon, 1961. Reprint, Éd. Gallimard, 1972.

———. *Naissance de la clinique.* PUF, 1963.

————. *Surveiller et punir.* Éd. Gallimard, 1975.

Fouché, Suzanne, *J'espérais d'un grand espoir.* Éd. du Cerf, 1981.

Fougeyrollas, Patrick. "Normalité et corps différents, regard sur l'intégration sociale des handicapés physiques." *Anthropologie et Sociétés* 2,
no. 2 (1978).

Fourquet, François, and Lion Murard. *Histoire de la psychiatrie de
secteur.* Éd. Recherches, 1980.

Fourquier, Guy. *Histoire économique et l'Occident médiéval.* Armand
Colin, 1979.

Freidson, Eliot. *Disability as Social Deviance: Sociology and Rehabilitation.* Washington, DC, American Sociological Association, 1965.

Fritz, Jean-Marie. *Le discours du fou au Moyen Âge, XIIe–XIIIe siècles,
étude comparée des discours littéraire, médical, juridique et théo-
logique de la folie.* PUF, 1992.

Gardou, Charles. *Handicaps, handicapés, le regard interrogé.* Érès,
1991.

Gateaux-Mennecier, Jacqueline. *La Débilité légère, une construction
idéologique,* preface by Éric Plaisance. Éd. du CNRS, 1990.

————. *Bourneville et l'enfance aliénée, l'humanisation du déficient mental au XIXe siècle,* preface by Roger Misès. Le Centurion, 1989. The
author also collaborated on the special issue of CTNERHI (1990) on the
historical evolution.

Gauchet, M. *Le Désenchantement du monde, une histoire politique de la
religion.* Éd. Gallimard, 1985.

Gauchet, Marcel, and Gladys Swain. *La pratique de l'esprit humain.
L'institution asilaire et la révolution démocratique.* Éd. Gallimard,
1980.

————. *Dialogue avec l'insensé.* Éd. Gallimard, 1994.

Geremek, Bronislaw. *La Potence ou la pitié, l'Europe et les pauvres du
Moyen Âge à nos jours.* Éd. Gallimard, 1986.

————. *Les Marginaux parisiens aux XIVe et XVe siècles.* Flammarion,
1976.

————. *Truands et misérables dans l'Europe moderne, 1350–1600.* Éd.
Gallimard, 1980.

Giami, Alain, G. Humert-Viveret, and D. Laval. *L'Ange et la Bête, représentation de la sexualité des handicapés mentaux par les parents et les
éducateurs.* CTNE-RHI, 1983.

Giami, in collaboration with Assouly-Piquet and Berthier-Vittoz. *La Figure fondamentale du handicap, représentations et figures fantas-
matiques.* MIRE-GERAL, 1988.

Gineste, Thierry. *Victor de l'Aveyron, dernier enfant sauvage, premier
enfant fou.* Le Sycomore, 1981.

Girard, René. *La Violence et le sacré.* Grasset, 1972.

———. *Des choses cachées depuis la fondation du monde.* Grasset, 1978.

Goffman, Erving. *Stigmate, les usages sociaux du handicap.* 1963. Reprint, Éd. de Minuit, 1975.

———. *Asiles—Études sur la condition sociale des malades mentaux.* Éd. de Minuit, 1968.

Goglin, Jean-Louis. *Les Misérables dans l'Occident médiéval.* Le Seuil, 1976.

Guillaume, Pierre. *Du Désespoir au salut: les tuberculeux aux XIXe–XXe siècles.* PUF, 1974.

"Handicap: identités, représentations, théories." *Sciences Sociales et Santé* 12 no. 1 (March 1994).

Heers, Jacques. *L'Occident aux XIVe et XVIe siècles, aspects économiques et sociaux.* PUF, 1973.

Henri, Pierre. *Les Aveugles et la société.* PUF, 1958.

Herzlich, Claudine. *Médecine, maladie, société.* Mouton, 1970.

———. *Santé et maladie, analyse d'une représentation sociale.* Mouton, 1984.

Imbert, Claude. *Les Hôpitaux en droit canonique.* Vrin, 1947.

Jacob, O. "Les Cités grecques et les blessés de guerre." *Mélanges G. Glotz,* 2 (1932).

Jodelet, Denise. *Folies et représentations sociales.* PUF, 1989.

Kanner, F. *A History of the Care and Study of Mental Retardation.* C. C. Thomas, 1964.

Kappler, Claude. *Le Monstre, pouvoir de l'imposture.* PUF, 1980.

Laharie, Muriel. *La Folie au Moyen Âge, XIe–XIIIe siècles.* Preface by Jacques Le Goff. Le Léopard d'Or, 1991.

Lallemand, L. *Histoire de la charité.* A. Picard et fils, 1902.

Lane, Harlan. *Quand l'esprit entend, histoire des sourds et muets.* Odile Jacob, 1991. Translated from *When the Mind Hears: A History of the Deaf.* Random House, 1984.

Lecouteux, Claude. *Les Monstres dans la pensée médiévale européenne.* Presse de l'Université de Paris-Sorbonne, 1993.

Le Goff, Jacques. *Pour un autre Moyen Âge, temps, travail et culture en Occident: 18 essais.* Éd. Gallimard, 1977.

———, ed. *La Nouvelle histoire.* Éd. Complexes, 1988.

Lenoir, René. *Les Exclus.* Le Seuil, 1974.

Léonard, Jacques. *La Médecine entre les pouvoirs et les savoirs, histoire intellectuelle et politique de la médecine française au XIXe siècle.* Aubier-Montaigne, 1981.

Lever, Maurice. *Le Sceptre et la Marotte, histoire des fous de cour.* Fayard, 1983.

———. *Les Invalides, deux siècles d'histoire.* Collectif, 1974.

Lévi-Strauss, Claude. *Anthropologie structurale.* 1958. Reprint, Plon, 1974.

———. *La Pensée sauvage.* Plon, 1962.

———. *Anthropologie structurale deux.* Plon, 1973.

———. *L'Impossible prison. Recherches sur le système pénitentiaire au XIXᵉ siècle,* ed. Michelle Perrot. Le Seuil, 1980.

Malson, Lucien. *Les Enfants sauvages, mythe et réalité.* 10/18. n.p., 1964.

Mausse, Marcel. *Sociologie et anthropologie.* PUF, 1950.

Mérian, J.B. *Sur le problème de Molyneux,* followed by *Mérian, Diderot et l'aveugle,* by Francine Markovits. Flammarion, 1984.

Michelet, André, and Gary Woodill. *Le Handicap mental, le fait social, le diagnostic, le traitement.* Delachaux et Niestlé, 1993.

Moi, Pierre Rivière, ayant égorgé ma mère, ma sœur et mon frère . . . Un cas de parricide au XIXᵉ siècle, edited by Michel Foucault. Éd. Gallimard/Julliard, 1973.

Mollat, Michel. *Les Pauvres au Moyen Âge, étude sociale.* Hachette, 1978.

Montes, Jean-François. *Travail—Infirme, des aveugles travailleurs aux travailleurs handicapés: genèse de la (re)mise au travail des infirmes.* Université de Paris I, DESS, 1989.

Morvan, J.S., and H. Paicheler, eds. *Représentations et handicaps: vers une clarification des concepts et des méthodes,* preface by D. Jodelet. CTNERHI et MIRE, 1990.

Moscovici, Serge. *La Psychanalyse, son image, son public.* PUF, 1981.

———. *Introduction à la psychologie sociale.* PUF, 1984.

Muel-Dreyfus, Francine. "L'école obligatoire et l'invention de l'enfance anormale." *Actes de la recherche en sciences sociales,* nos. 32–33 (1975).

Murphy, Robert. *Vivre à corps perdu.* Plon, Terre Humaine, 1990. Translated from *The Body Silent: A Journey into Paralysis.* Henry Holt, 1987.

Oé, Kenzaruro. *Une affaire personnelle.* Stock, 1968.

———. *Dites-nous comment survivre à notre folie.* Éd. Gallimard, 1982.

Paicheler, Henri; Béatrice Beaufils, Claudette Edrei. *La Represésentation sociale de la personnalité handicapée physique.* Rapport de Recherche, CTNERHI, 1983.

Paré, Ambroise. *Des Monstres et prodiges,* ed., Jean Céard. Droz, 1971.

Pélicier, Yves, and Guy Thuillier. *Édouard Seguin, l'instituteur des idiots.* Économica, 1980.

Paugam, Serge, ed. *L'Exclusion, l'état des savoirs.* Éd. La Découverte, 1996.

Peter, Jean-Pierre, and Michel Cazenave. *L'imaginaire des maladies dans J. Le Goff et al.*, Histoire et Imaginaire. Radio-France-Poésis, 1986.

Pigeaud, Jackie. *La Maladie de l'âme. Étude sur la relation de l'âme et du corps dans la tradition médico-philosophique antique.* Les Belles Lettres, 1981.

———. *Folie et cures de la folie chez les médecins de l'antiquité gréco-romaine. La manie.* Les Belles Lettres, 1987.

Pinell, Patrice. "L'école obligatoire et les recherches en psychopédagogie au début du XXᵉ siècle." *Cahiers Internationaux de Sociologie* 63 (1977).

Pinell, Patrice, and M. Zafiropoulos. *Un siècle d'échecs scolaires (1882–1982).* Éd. de l'Atelier, Éd. Ouvrières, 1983.

Postel, Jacques, and Claude Quétel, eds. *Nouvelle histoire de la psychiatrie.* Éd. Private, 1983. Dunod, 1994.

Presneau, Jean-René. *L'idée de surdité et l'éducation des enfants sourds et muets, en France et en Espagne du XVIᵉ au XVIIIᵉ siècle.* Ph.D. diss., EHESS, Paris, 1980.

Prost, Antoine. *Les Anciens combattants et la société française, 1914–1939.* Presses de la Fondation Nationale des Sciences Politiques, 1977.

Quétel, Claude, and P. Morel. *Les Fous et leurs médecines de la Renaissance au XXᵉ siècle.* Hachette, 1979.

———. *Médecines de la folie.* Hachette, 1985.

Raynaud, Philippe. "L'éducation spécialisée en France (1882–1982)." *Esprit*, nos. 5, 7–8 (1982).

Roger, Jacques. *Les Sciences de la vie dans la pensée française au XVIIIᵉ siècle.* 1963. Reprint, Albin Michel, 1993.

Saint Francis of Assisi. *Documents: écrits et premières biographies*, ed. Théophile Desbonnets and Damien Vorreux. Éd. Franciscaines, 1968.

Saladin, Monique, Alain Casanova, and Umberto Vidali. *Le Regard des autres.* Preface by Michel Fardeau. Fleurus, 1990.

Sassie, Philippe. *Du bon usage des pauvres. Histoire d'un thème politique, XVIᵉ–XXᵉ siècle.* Fayard, 1990.

Sausse, Simone. *Le Miroir brisé, l'enfant handicapé, sa famille et le psychanalyste.* Calmann-Lévy, 1996.

Schimitt, Jean-Claude. "Anthropologie historique." *Dictionnaire de l'ethnologie et de l'anthropologie*, ed. P. Bonte and M. Izard. PUF, 1991.

Semélaigne, René. *Aliénation mentale dans l'Antiquité.* 1869.

Simon, B. *Mind and Mindness in Ancient Greece.* Cornell University Press, 1979.

Simondon, Gilbert. *L'Individu et sa genèse physico-biologique.* PUF, 1964.

Starobinski, Jean. *Histoire du traitement de la mélancolie des origines à nos jours.* n.p., 1965.

Stiker, Henri-Jacques. "De la métaphore au modèle: l'anthropologie du handicap." *Cahiers Ethnologiques* (University of Bordeaux), no. 13 (1991).

———. "Handicap, handicapé." In *Handicap et inadaptation. Fragments pour une histoire. Notions et acteurs.* Alter, 1996.

———. "Les catégories organisatrices de l'infirmité." In *Handicap vécu, évalué.* La Pensée Sauvage, 1987.

"Les Ménines, image de pouvoir, dérision du pouvoir." *Revue Esprit,* no. 11 (1985).

———. *Culture brisée, culture à naître.* Aubier, 1979.

———. "La révolution française et les infirmes." In *Les Acquis de la Révolution Française pour les personnes handicapées de 1789 à nos jours.* Université Paris X–Nanterre, 1991.

Stiker, H. J., M. Viral, and C. Barral, eds. *Handicap et inadaptation, fragments pour une histoire, notions et acteurs.* Alter, 1996.

Swain, Gladys. *Le sujet de la folie. Naissance de la psychiatrie.* Éd. Privat, 1977.

———. "Une logique de l'inclusion: les infirmes du signe." *Revue Esprit,* (May 1982). (See also Gauchet, Marcel.)

Talbot, M. E. *Édouard Seguin: A Study of an Educational Approach to the Treatment of Mentally Defective Children.* Teachers College Press, 1964.

Tomlinson, Sally. *A Sociology of Special Education.* Routledge and Kegan Paul, 1982.

Touati, François-Olivier. "Lèpre, lépreux et léproseries dans la province ecclésiastique de Sens jusqu'au milieu du quatorzième siècle." Master's thesis, Université Panthéon-Sorbonne, Paris I, 1991. Part of this work, devoted exclusively to geography appeared as *Archives de la lèpre, atlas des léproseries entre Loire et Marne au Moyen Âge.* CTHS, 1996.

Turpin, Pierre. "La lutte contre l'assistance pendant les années 1970." In *De l'infirmité au handicap: jalons historiques.* Les cahiers du CTNERHI, handicaps et inadaptations, no. 50 (April–June 1990).

Veil, Claude. *Handicap et société.* Nouvelle Bibliothèque Scientifique, ed. Fernand Braudel. Flammarion, 1968.

Verdes-Leroux, Jeannine. *Le Travail social.* Éd. de Minuit, 1978.

Vernant, Jean-Pierre. "*Ambiguïté et Renversement. Sur la structure énigmatique d'Œdipe-roi.*" In *Échanges et Communications. Mélanges offerts à Claude Lévi-Strauss* 2 (1970), 1253–79. Reprinted in J.-P. Vernant and P. Vidal-Naquet, *Œdipe et ses mythes* (Éd. Complexes, 1988).

————. "Le tyran boiteux, d'Œdipe à Périandre." In *Le Temps de la réflexion*. Éd. Gallimard, 1981. Reprinted in *Œdipe et ses mythes*.

Vernant, Jean-Pierre, and Marcel Detienne. *Les ruses de l'intelligence, la métis des grecs*. Flammarion, 1974.

Veyne, Paul. *Comment on écrit l'histoire suivi de Foucault révolutionne l'histoire*. Le Seuil, 1978.

Vial, Monique. *Les enfants anormaux à l'école. Aux origines de l'éducation spécialisée, 1882–1909*, preface by Antoine Prost. Armand Colin, 1990. Monique Vial collaborated on *De l'infirmité au handicap, jalons historiques* and *Fragments pour une histoire*.

Vigarello, Georges. *Le Corps redressé: histoire d'un pouvoir pédagogique*. J.-P. Delarge, 1978.

Villey, Pierre. *L'Aveugle dans le monde des voyants. Essai de sociologie*. Flammarion, 1927.

————. *Le Monde des aveugles*. 1918.

Vincent, Bernard. Presentation of *Les Marginaux et les exclus dans l'histoire*. Cahiers Jussieu/5 Université Paris 7, 10/18, 1979.

Saint Vincent de Paul. *Œuvres complètes*. Éd. Coste, n.d.

Wacjman, Claude. "Désiré Magloire Bourneville dans le grand centenaire de la Révolution." *L'Évolution Psychiatrique* 55, no. 1 (January–March 1990).

————. *L'Enfance inadaptée, anthologie de textes fondamentaux*. Éd. Privat, 1993.

Werner, H. *History of the Problem of Deaf-Mutism until the Seventeenth Century*. Gustav Fisher, 1932.

Weygnad, Zina. *Les causes de la cécité et les soins oculaires en France au début du XIXe siècle (1800–1815)*. CTNERHI, n.d.

Wolf, Hans-Walter. *Anthropologie de l'Ancien Testament*. Labor et Fides, 1974.

Woodill, Gary. *Bibliographie signalétique, Histoire des handicaps et inadaptations, Thematic Bibliography on the history of disabilities and social problems*. CTNERHI, 1988.

Zafiropoulos, M. *Les Arriérés, de l'asile à l'usine*. Payot, 1969.

Zazzo, René. *Les Débilités mentales*. Colin, 1969.